Internal Medicine Evidence

The Practice-Changing Studies

EDITORS

Joshua M. Liao, MD
Staff Physician
Department of Medicine
University of Pennsylvania School
  of Medicine
Philadelphia, Pennsylvania

Zahir Kanjee, MD, MPH
Hospitalist
Beth Israel Deaconess Medical Center
Instructor in Medicine
Harvard Medical School
Boston, Massachusetts

SPECIAL EDITORS

Joel T. Katz, MD
Joseph Loscalzo, MD, PhD

SERIES EDITORS

Emily L. Aaronson, MD
Erik L. Antonsen, MD, PhD
Arjun K. Venkatesh, MD, MBA, MHS

SECTION EDITOR

Luis Ticona, MD, MPP

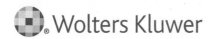

Philadelphia • Baltimore • New York • London
Buenos Aires • Hong Kong • Sydney • Tokyo

Executive Editor: Rebecca S. Gaertner
Senior Development Editor: Kristina Oberle
Marketing Manager: Rachel Mante Leung
Production Project Manager: David Saltzberg
Design Coordinator: Holly Reid McLaughlin
Manufacturing Coordinator: Beth Welsh
Prepress Vendor: Aptara, Inc.

Printed in China

Library of Congress Cataloging-in-Publication Data
Names: Liao, Joshua M., editor. | Kanjee, Zahir, editor. | Katz, Joel T., editor. | Loscalzo, Joseph, editor.
Title: Internal medicine evidence : the practice-changing studies / editors, Joshua M. Liao, Zahir Kanjee ; special editors, Joel T. Katz, Joseph Loscalzo.
Description: Philadelphia : Wolters Kluwer, [2017] | Includes bibliographical references and index.
Identifiers: LCCN 2017000194 | ISBN 9781496343550 (paperback)
Subjects: | MESH: Internal Medicine | Evidence-Based Medicine | Clinical Trials as Topic | Handbooks
Classification: LCC RC46 | NLM WB 39 | DDC 616—dc23
LC record available at https://lccn.loc.gov/2017000194

CCS0317

To my wife (Geraldine), daughter (Abigail), brother (Caleb), and parents (Sandra and Samuel), for being foundations of good in my life and showing me the importance of aligning knowledge with practice in both work and life.

Joshua M. Liao, MD

To my parents, Aziz and Amina, for supporting me at every step; to my wife, Kendra, and daughter, Roya, for sharing me with this project; and to my teachers – two of whom are special editors on this volume – who have modeled and reinforced the links between understanding clinical evidence and practicing clinical excellence.

Zahir Kanjee, MD, MPH

CONTRIBUTORS

Viswatej Avutu, MD
Resident in Medicine and Pediatrics
Brigham and Women's Hospital/Boston
  Children's Hospital
Clinical Fellow in Medicine
Harvard Medical School
Boston, Massachusetts

Anthony Carnicelli, MD
Resident in Medicine
Brigham and Women's Hospital
Clinical Fellow in Medicine
Harvard Medical School
Boston, Massachusetts

Alexandra Charrow, MD, MBE
Resident in Medicine and Dermatology
Brigham and Women's Hospital/Harvard
  Combined Dermatology Residency
  Program
Clinical Fellow in Medicine
Harvard Medical School
Boston, Massachusetts

Ersilia M. DeFilippis, MD
Resident in Medicine
Brigham and Women's Hospital
Clinical Fellow in Medicine
Harvard Medical School
Boston, Massachusetts

Kristin Castillo Farias, MD
Primary Care Physician in Internal Medicine
  and Pediatrics
Departments of Medicine and Pediatrics
Cambridge Health Alliance
Cambridge, Massachusetts

Amy O. Flaster, MD, MBA
Resident in Medicine
Brigham and Women's Hospital
Clinical Fellow in Medicine
Harvard Medical School
Boston, Massachusetts

Michael C. Honigberg, MD, MPP
Resident in Medicine
Brigham and Women's Hospital
Clinical Fellow in Medicine
Harvard Medical School
Boston, Massachusetts

Michelle Jose-Kampfner, MD
Resident in Medicine
Brigham and Women's Hospital
Clinical Fellow in Medicine
Harvard Medical School
Boston, Massachusetts

Erik H. Knelson, MD, PhD
Resident in Medicine
Brigham and Women's Hospital
Clinical Fellow in Medicine
Harvard Medical School
Boston, Massachusetts

Vivek T. Kulkarni, MD, MHS
Resident in Medicine
Brigham and Women's Hospital
Clinical Fellow in Medicine
Harvard Medical School
Boston, Massachusetts

Melissa G. Lechner, MD, PhD
Resident in Medicine and Pediatrics
Brigham and Women's Hospital/Boston
    Children's Hospital
Clinical Fellow in Medicine
Harvard Medical School
Boston, Massachusetts

Jessica Lee-Pancoast, MD, MHS
Resident in Medicine
Brigham and Women's Hospital
Clinical Fellow in Medicine
Harvard Medical School
Boston, Massachusetts

Gabriel B. Loeb, MD, PhD
Resident in Medicine
Brigham and Women's Hospital
Clinical Fellow in Medicine
Harvard Medical School
Boston, Massachusetts

Nadim Mahmud, MD, MPH, MS
Resident in Medicine
Brigham and Women's Hospital
Clinical Fellow in Medicine
Harvard Medical School
Boston, Massachusetts

Anish Mehta, MD, MPP
Resident in Medicine
Brigham and Women's Hospital
Clinical Fellow in Medicine
Harvard Medical School
Boston, Massachusetts

Daniel O'Neil, MD
Resident in Medicine
Brigham and Women's Hospital
Clinical Fellow in Medicine
Harvard Medical School
Boston, Massachusetts

Neelam A. Phadke, MD
Resident in Medicine and Pediatrics
Brigham and Women's Hospital/Boston
    Children's Hospital
Clinical Fellow in Medicine
Harvard Medical School
Boston, Massachusetts

Sarah E. Post, MD
Resident in Medicine
Brigham and Women's Hospital
Clinical Fellow in Medicine
Harvard Medical School
Boston, Massachusetts

Elizabeth A. Richey, MD, MS
Resident in Medicine
Brigham and Women's Hospital
Clinical Fellow in Medicine
Harvard Medical School
Boston, Massachusetts

Julia Rudolf, MD
Resident in Medicine
Brigham and Women's Hospital
Clinical Fellow in Medicine
Harvard Medical School
Boston, Massachusetts

Luis M. Ticona, MD, MPP
Health Policy and Management Fellow
Massachusetts General Physician
    Organization
Instructor in Medicine
Harvard Medical School
Boston, Massachusetts

Mounica Vallurupalli, MD
Resident in Medicine
Brigham and Women's Hospital
Clinical Fellow in Medicine
Harvard Medical School
Boston, Massachusetts

Anubodh Varshney, MD
Resident in Medicine
Brigham and Women's Hospital
Clinical Fellow in Medicine
Harvard Medical School
Boston, Massachusetts

PREFACE

In this volume, we aspired to select, summarize, and contextualize 100 of the most practice-changing articles in the field of internal medicine. As practicing clinicians, medical educators, and lifelong learners, we felt particularly drawn to the challenge of exploring how evidence guides clinical choices. In doing so, we hope to shed light on the strengths and weaknesses, clinical and historical context, and impacts and caveats of important research studies that underlie common and challenging clinical decisions.

Our goal was to select articles representing the diverse subspecialty areas within internal medicine, employing a systematic approach that began by drawing upon article aggregators, clinical compendia, evidence-based medicine resources, citation trackers, as well as our own clinical knowledge base. Within each subspecialty, we then identified common topics and clinical conditions of importance to internists. Articles identified through these processes were then evaluated within a larger context through a review of prevailing clinical guidelines and relevant critiques, editorials, correspondence, and follow-up studies. Additionally, we solicited input from clinicians affiliated with Harvard Medical School, both to refine our list as well as review content once written.

Our article selection process incorporated two strategic choices. First, we balanced the desire to achieve breadth of covered topics against the imperative of representing the strongest level of evidence possible. This led us to favor prospective, randomized trials over quasiexperimental or descriptive retrospective studies whenever possible, and at times, omitting topics not because they were unimportant, but because strong evidence was lacking. Second, we prioritized articles that represented fundamental, rather than incremental, shifts in practice. This approach, for example, led us to prioritize the earliest, paradigm-shifting and practice-changing articles demonstrating the benefit of direct oral anticoagulants over warfarin in atrial fibrillation and venous thromboembolism, rather than subsequent studies comparing the incremental effects of different direct oral agents.

Despite these measures, we recognize the inherent challenges of integrating multiple considerations (e.g., topical inclusiveness, strength of evidence, disease prevalence, and current and historical clinical interest) to arrive at a single list of 100 articles, particularly when entire volumes could be written for individual subspecialties within internal medicine. While there is certainly room for challenging our choices, we hope there is consensus that the analysis of these 100 articles highlights and fuels discussion about how evidence impacts clinical practice.

Ultimately, we hope that by strengthening the connection between evidence and clinical practice, this volume will be a valuable contribution to all those involved in internal medicine, including trainees and clinicians at all stages of their careers. We also hope that you enjoy reading it as much as we did editing it.

Joshua M. Liao, MD
Zahir Kanjee, MD, MPH

ACKNOWLEDGMENTS

We are indebted to a number of people who helped make this book possible. We are grateful to the Brigham and Women's Hospital Internal Medicine Residency as well as faculty in the Department of Medicine who helped with the article selection process. We would like to especially thank the following clinicians affiliated with Harvard Medical School for their content review: Drs. Philippe Armand, Rebecca Baron, Nancy Berliner, Paul Dellaripa, Christopher Fanta, Ann LaCasce, Bruce Levy, Dan Longo, Robert Mayer, Ronald McCaffrey, Jennifer Nayor, Beth Overmoyer, Juan Carl Pallais, Aric Parnes, Kunal Patel, Scott Schissel, Sunita Sharma, Alice Sheridan, Robert Soiffer, David Steensma, Christopher Sweeney, and Amanda Redig.

Most importantly, we acknowledge and salute all of the patients who volunteered to participate in these studies, along with those who will continue to do so in future studies, each of whom allow medicine to continually move forward.

CONTENTS

SECTION 1: CARDIOLOGY
Section Editor: Joshua M. Liao

SECTION 2: CRITICAL CARE
Section Editor: Zahir Kanjee

SECTION 3: ENDOCRINOLOGY
Section Editor: Joshua M. Liao

SECTION 4: GASTROENTEROLOGY
Section Editor: Zahir Kanjee

SECTION 5: HEMATOLOGY
Section Editor: Luis Ticona

SECTION 6: INFECTIOUS DISEASES
Section Editor: Zahir Kanjee

SECTION 7: NEPHROLOGY
Section Editor: Luis Ticona

SECTION 8: ONCOLOGY
Section Editor: Luis Ticona

SECTION 9: PULMONOLOGY
Section Editors: Zahir Kanjee, Joshua M. Liao

SECTION 10: RHEUMATOLOGY
Section Editor: Joshua M. Liao

CHAPTER 1

RATE VERSUS RHYTHM CONTROL IN ATRIAL FIBRILLATION: THE AFFIRM TRIAL

Anubodh Varshney

A Comparison of Rate Control and Rhythm Control in Patients With Atrial Fibrillation
Wyse DG, Waldo AL, DiMarco JP, et al. *N Engl J Med.* 2002;347(23):1825–1833

BACKGROUND

Prior to this study, the optimal strategy for managing atrial fibrillation (AF) was uncertain. The preferred therapy for reducing morbidity and mortality had been maintenance of sinus rhythm by cardioversion and/or antiarrhythmic medications ("rhythm control"). However, AF is poorly responsive to antiarrhythmics, which can also have significant adverse effects. The long-term impact of the alternative strategy – maintaining a ventricular rate with atrioventricular nodal blocking medications ("rate control") – was also unknown.

OBJECTIVES

To compare the effects of long-term treatment with rate control versus rhythm control in patients with AF.

METHODS

Randomized controlled trial at 213 clinical sites in the United States and Canada between 1995 and 1999.

Patients

4,060 patients. Inclusion criteria included age ≥65 years (or with risk factors for stroke or death if <65 years) and AF that was likely to be recurrent, cause illness or death, and warrant long-term treatment. Exclusion criteria included contraindication to anticoagulation and inability to undergo trials of ≥2 medications in either arm.

Interventions

Rhythm control (using oral class I and III antiarrhythmics, with cardioversion as necessary based on physician judgment, to maintain sinus rhythm) versus rate control (using beta blockers, calcium channel blockers, or digoxin to maintain goal resting heart rate <80 bpm and <110 bpm during 6-minute walk test). All patients were anticoagulated with warfarin (goal INR 2.0 to 3.0). Those in the rhythm-control group could discontinue anticoagulation if sinus rhythm was maintained for ≥4 weeks.

Outcomes

The primary outcome was overall mortality. The composite secondary outcome was death, disabling stroke, disabling anoxic encephalopathy, major bleeding, or cardiac arrest.

KEY RESULTS
- At 5 years, there were no statistically significant differences in the rate of overall mortality between the two groups (25.9% in rate-control group vs. 26.7% in rhythm-control group, $p = 0.08$).
- There were no statistically significant differences with respect to the composite secondary outcome (32.7% vs. 32.0%, $p = 0.33$).
- Rates of pulmonary events, gastrointestinal events, bradycardia, QTc prolongation prompting drug discontinuation, and hospitalization were all higher in the rhythm-control group ($p < 0.001$ for each).
- For both rate- and rhythm-control groups, the majority of strokes occurred after discontinuation of warfarin or when INR was subtherapeutic.

STUDY CONCLUSIONS
Management of AF with a rhythm-control strategy offers no survival advantage over a rate-control strategy. Rate control is also associated with a lower risk of adverse drug effects.

COMMENTARY

AFFIRM was pivotal for comparing these two strategies and demonstrating that rhythm control using a range of antiarrhythmics did not exhibit the presumed benefits over rate control and actually led to increased rates of hospitalization and adverse events. It also showed that anticoagulation should be continued in high-risk patients, even when sinus rhythm is restored. Caveats include lack of generalizability to younger patients without stroke risk factors (e.g., those with "lone" AF) or those with symptomatic AF. AFFIRM contributed to the adoption of rate control in clinical practice, and 2014 AHA/ACC/HRS guidelines recommend it as a reasonable option for patients with asymptomatic AF.

Question
Is it reasonable to treat elderly patients with recurrent, asymptomatic AF with a rate-control strategy?

Answer
Yes, rate control is associated with a lower risk of adverse drug effects compared to rhythm control.

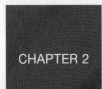

CHAPTER 2

ANGIOPLASTY VERSUS STREPTOKINASE IN MYOCARDIAL INFARCTION

Michael C. Honigberg

A Comparison of Immediate Coronary Angioplasty With Intravenous Streptokinase in Acute Myocardial Infarction

Zijlstra F, de Boer MJ, Hoorntje JC, Reiffers S, Reiber JH, Suryapranata H. *N Engl J Med.* 1993;328(10):680–684

BACKGROUND

Prior to 1993, systemic intravenous thrombolysis, heparin, and aspirin constituted standard management of acute ST-elevation myocardial infarction (STEMI). Angioplasty had not shown benefit as an adjunctive treatment for revascularization, except as "rescue" therapy in infarct-related arteries that failed to reperfuse after thrombolysis. However, the effect of immediate, nonrescue angioplasty had not been directly compared to thrombolysis in large prospective studies.

OBJECTIVES

To compare immediate angioplasty and intravenous thrombolysis in acute STEMI.

METHODS

Randomized controlled trial at a single center in the Netherlands between 1990 and 1992.

Patients

142 patients. Inclusion criteria included age ≤75 years, ischemic chest pain ≥30 minutes in duration, ST-segment elevations ≥1 mm in ≥2 contiguous ECG leads, presentation ≤6 hours from symptom onset (or ≤24 hours if ongoing ischemic symptoms), and no contraindication to fibrinolysis.

Interventions

Immediate angioplasty (mean admission-to-balloon time = 61 minutes) versus intravenous streptokinase infusion (mean admission-to-infusion time = 30 minutes). All patients received aspirin, intravenous heparin, and a nitroglycerin infusion titrated to SBP 110 mm Hg.

Outcomes

The outcomes evaluated were recurrent ischemia (stable angina, unstable angina, and recurrent MI) prior to discharge, vessel patency as assessed by coronary angiography, and left ventricular ejection fraction (LVEF). Complications included death, stroke, bleeding (intercerebral bleeding or bleeding necessitating blood transfusion), heart failure, and need for bypass surgery.

KEY RESULTS

- Patients undergoing angioplasty experienced less recurrent ischemia (9% vs. 38%, $p < 0.001$) and recurrent infarction (0% vs. 13%, $p = 0.003$).
- The angioplasty group also had more favorable mean LVEF (51% vs. 45%, $p = 0.004$) prior to hospital discharge and higher rates of vessel patency (91% vs. 68%, $p = 0.001$).
- There were no statistically significant differences in complication rates ($p > 0.05$ for all).

STUDY CONCLUSIONS

Among patients presenting with acute STEMI, immediate angioplasty was associated with less recurrent ischemia and infarction, a higher rate of coronary artery patency, less severe residual stenosis, and better left ventricular function compared to thrombolysis with intravenous streptokinase.

COMMENTARY

Although much has changed in the management of acute coronary syndrome (ACS) since 1993, this study helped shift the treatment paradigm for STEMI from thrombolysis toward percutaneous coronary intervention (PCI) and justify resource investments to increase local PCI availability. Together with other studies and the advent of coronary stents, these results have led to a new standard of care, and the 2013 ACCF/AHA STEMI guidelines recommend PCI with stent placement as the preferred treatment strategy, with thrombolysis generally reserved for cases when prompt intervention is not possible (e.g., time from first medical contact to intervention at a PCI-capable center >2 hours).

Question

Is immediate angioplasty preferred over thrombolysis in the treatment of patients with acute STEMI?

Answer

Yes, compared to thrombolysis, angioplasty reduces recurrent ischemia and infarction and achieves superior vessel patency and ventricular function, although PCI with stent placement is now the standard of care.

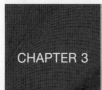

FIRST-STEP ANTIHYPERTENSIVE THERAPY: THE ALLHAT TRIAL

CHAPTER 3

Nadim Mahmud

Major Outcomes in High-Risk Hypertensive Patients Randomized to Angiotensin-Converting Enzyme Inhibitor or Calcium Channel Blocker vs. Diuretic: The Antihypertensive and Lipid-Lowering Treatment to Prevent Heart Attack Trial (ALLHAT)

ALLHAT Officers and Coordinators for the ALLHAT Collaborative Research Group. *JAMA*. 2002;288(23):2981–2997

BACKGROUND

Early trials had demonstrated the cardiovascular disease (CVD) benefits of controlling hypertension with beta blockers and thiazide diuretics. Subsequently, several new antihypertensive classes were developed, including angiotensin-converting enzyme (ACE) inhibitors and calcium channel blockers (CCBs). Prior to this study, these medications had been tested against placebo but were never compared head to head as initial antihypertensive therapy.

OBJECTIVES

To compare the effects of ACE inhibitors, CCBs, and thiazides in high-risk hypertensive patients.

METHODS

Randomized, controlled, double-blind trial in 623 North American institutions between 1994 and 2002.

Patients

33,357 patients. Inclusion criteria included age ≥55 years with stage 1 or 2 hypertension and ≥1 coronary heart disease (CHD) risk factor (recent myocardial infarction [MI] or stroke, left ventricular hypertrophy, smoking, type 2 diabetes, high-density lipoprotein cholesterol <35 mg/dL, or other atherosclerotic CVD). Exclusion criteria included left ventricular ejection fraction <35% and heart failure (HF) treatment or hospitalizations.

Interventions

Lisinopril versus amlodipine versus chlorthalidone as the initial antihypertensive agent, titrated to a goal BP <140/90 mm Hg. Previous BP agents were stopped, and atenolol, clonidine, or reserpine could be added as additional open-label agents to achieve the BP goal.

Outcomes

The primary outcome was combined incidence of fatal CHD or nonfatal MI. Secondary outcomes included all-cause mortality and stroke.

KEY RESULTS

- There was no difference in the 6-year rate of the primary outcome between chlorthalidone and amlodipine (11.5% vs. 11.3%, $p = 0.65$) or chlorthalidone and lisinopril (11.5% vs. 11.4%, $p = 0.81$).
- There was no difference in 6-year rates of all-cause mortality between chlorthalidone and amlodipine (17.3% vs. 16.8%, $p = 0.20$) or between chlorthalidone and lisinopril (17.3% vs. 17.2%, $p = 0.90$).
- Compared to the chlorthalidone group, the lisinopril group had a higher rate of HF (8.7% vs. 7.7%, $p < 0.001$) and stroke (6.3% vs. 5.6%, $p = 0.02$) at 6 years.
- Compared to those receiving chlorthalidone, black patients receiving lisinopril were more likely to suffer stroke (RR 1.40, 95% CI 1.17–1.68).
- Compared to the chlorthalidone group, the amlodipine group had a higher 6-year rate of HF (10.2% vs. 7.7%, $p < 0.001$).

STUDY CONCLUSIONS

Chlorthalidone was more effective than lisinopril or amlodipine in preventing one or more types of CVD.

COMMENTARY

By showing that thiazides can be more effective in preventing CVD than the other more expensive agents tested, ALLHAT shifted clinical practice toward thiazides as the initial pharmacotherapy for hypertension. Caveats include the fact that the lisinopril group did not achieve the same degree of BP lowering as the chlorthalidone group and the uncertainty about extrapolating these results to different thiazides (e.g., from chlorthalidone to hydrochlorothiazide). Based in part on the ALLHAT results, thiazides remain a first-line option for hypertension in the 7th and 8th Joint National Committee guidelines.

Question

Is chlorthalidone a reasonable first-step BP medication?

Answer

Yes, chlorthalidone is equivalent to lisinopril and amlodipine with respect to fatal CHD or nonfatal MI, and can be superior in decreasing major forms of CVD (HF and stroke). However, patient comorbidities may dictate selection of another first agent.

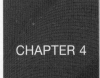

CHAPTER 4

HEART FAILURE TREATMENT FOR AFRICAN AMERICANS: THE A-HeFT TRIAL

Michael C. Honigberg

Combination of Isosorbide Dinitrate and Hydralazine in Blacks With Heart Failure

Taylor AL, Ziesche S, Yancy C, et al. *N Engl J Med*. 2004;351(20):2049–2057

BACKGROUND

Though earlier studies had demonstrated the benefit of treating heart failure (HF) with combined nitrate and hydralazine therapy, its long-term effect among patients receiving neurohormonal blockade (e.g., beta blockers, ACE inhibitors, and mineralocorticoid receptor antagonists) was unknown. Retrospective data also suggested that black patients might have a particularly favorable response to this combination therapy.

OBJECTIVES

To evaluate the efficacy of a fixed-dose combination of hydralazine and isosorbide dinitrate in HF patients who self-identify as black.

METHODS

Randomized, placebo-controlled, double-blind trial at 161 sites in the United States between 2001 and 2004.

Patients

1,050 patients. Inclusion criteria included age >18 years, self-identified black race, New York Heart Association (NYHA) class III–IV HF, left ventricular ejection fraction (LVEF) ≤35% or <45% with LV dilatation, and receipt of standard HF therapy for ≥3 months. Exclusion criteria included recent acute coronary syndrome, stroke, cardiac surgery, cardiac arrest, or inotrope requirement, symptomatic hypotension, and valvular or infiltrative heart disease.

Interventions

Combination therapy (tablet containing 37.5 mg hydralazine and 20 mg isosorbide dinitrate 3 times daily, uptitrated to 2 tablets 3 times daily as tolerated) versus placebo. All patients received standard HF therapy and were followed for up to 18 months (mean follow-up 10 months).

Outcomes

The primary outcome was a composite score comprising all-cause mortality, time to first HF hospitalization, and change in quality of life. Secondary outcomes included individual components of the primary outcome, death from cardiovascular causes, and HF hospitalizations.

KEY RESULTS

- The trial was terminated early per protocol due to greater mortality in patients receiving placebo (10.2% vs. 6.2%, $p = 0.02$).
- Patients receiving combination therapy achieved more favorable primary composite scores (-0.1 ± 1.9 vs. -0.5 ± 2.0, $p = 0.01$).
- Those receiving combination therapy were less likely to experience a first HF hospitalization (16.4% vs. 24.4%, $p = 0.001$) and reported greater improvement in quality of life at 6 months.

STUDY CONCLUSIONS

Among blacks with advanced HF, the addition of hydralazine and isosorbide dinitrate to standard therapy reduces morbidity and mortality.

COMMENTARY

A-HeFT was important for demonstrating the benefit of combination therapy among a group that bears a disproportionate share of HF morbidity and mortality. Caveats that limit generalizability include assessment of race by self-report rather than another potentially more objective manner and enrollment of few patients with class IV HF (~5%). Additionally, the side-effect profile (e.g., headache, dizziness), frequent dosing, and large pill burden – which is often further compounded by use of separate, rather than combination, pills – may limit adherence in real-world practice. Based largely on A-HeFT, the 2013 ACC/AHA heart failure guidelines recommend the use of combined nitrate/hydralazine in black patients with NYHA III–IV HF with reduced LVEF.

Question

Should patients who self-identify as black and exhibit severe symptoms from HF with reduced LVEF receive combined hydralazine and nitrate therapy?

Answer

Yes, when added to other medical therapy, the combination decreases HF morbidity and mortality.

| CHAPTER 5 | DUAL ANTIPLATELET THERAPY IN NON–ST-ELEVATION ACS: THE CURE TRIAL |

Anubodh Varshney

Effects of Clopidogrel in Addition to Aspirin in Patients With Acute Coronary Syndromes Without ST-Segment Elevation

Yusuf S, Zhao F, Mehta SR, et al. *N Engl J Med*. 2001;345(7):494–502

BACKGROUND

Prior to this study, the advent of percutaneous transluminal coronary angioplasty (PTCA), glycoprotein IIb/IIIa inhibitors, and early anticoagulation had reduced morbidity and mortality associated with acute coronary syndrome (ACS). However, patients remained at high risk for recurrent myocardial infarction (MI). Despite knowledge that adding a platelet inhibitor such as clopidogrel to aspirin for a short time decreased recurrent MI in patients undergoing angioplasty with stenting, the long-term safety and efficacy of such dual antiplatelet therapy (DAPT) remained unknown.

OBJECTIVES

To determine the safety and efficacy of the early and long-term use of clopidogrel plus aspirin in patients with non–ST-elevation ACS (NSTE-ACS).

METHODS

Randomized, double-blind, placebo-controlled trial at 482 medical centers in 28 countries between 1998 and 2000.

Patients

12,562 patients. Inclusion criteria included hospitalization ≤24 hours after onset of NSTE-ACS with evidence of ischemia from either electrocardiography or serum cardiac biomarkers. Exclusion criteria included contraindications to antithrombotic therapy, use of oral anticoagulants, high risk for bleeding, severe heart failure, coronary revascularization within the previous 3 months, or recent glycoprotein IIb/IIIa inhibitor exposure.

Interventions

Clopidogrel (300 mg loading dose followed by 75 mg daily) versus placebo for 3 to 12 months. All patients also received aspirin (75 to 325 mg daily).

Outcomes

The two primary outcomes were the composite of death from cardiovascular causes, nonfatal MI or stroke, and the composite of the first primary outcome or refractory ischemia. Secondary outcomes included in-hospital severe ischemia, heart failure, and need for revascularization. Safety outcomes were life-threatening, major, or minor bleeding complications.

KEY RESULTS

- The composite of death from cardiovascular causes, nonfatal MI, or stroke was lower in the clopidogrel group (9.3% vs. 11.4%, RR 0.80, 95% CI 0.72–0.90, $p < 0.001$).
- The composite of the first primary outcome or refractory ischemia was lower in the clopidogrel group (16.5% vs. 18.8%, RR 0.86, 95% CI 0.79–0.94, $p < 0.001$) with risk reductions beginning by 24 hours after randomization and lasting through 12 months.
- Major (3.7% vs. 2.7%, $p = 0.001$) and minor (5.1% vs. 2.4%, $p < 0.001$) bleeding were more common in the clopidogrel group, but there were no differences in fatal bleeding, bleeding requiring surgery, or hemorrhagic stroke.

STUDY CONCLUSIONS

The addition of clopidogrel to aspirin has beneficial effects in patients presenting with NSTE-ACS, but is also associated with increased bleeding risk.

COMMENTARY

CURE was the first large trial to demonstrate the anti-ischemic benefits of DAPT in patients with ACS. Caveats include a lower fraction of patients undergoing PTCA than in subsequent clinical practice, and results should be interpreted in view of clopidogrel's potential to delay coronary artery bypass graft surgery (CABG). Nonetheless, subsequent studies have supported the role of clopidogrel or other antiplatelet agents such as prasugrel and ticagrelor in ACS management. Collectively, this work has led to routine use of DAPT and its incorporation into both the 2012 ACCF/AHA guidelines for the management of NSTE-ACS and 2013 ACCF/AHA guidelines for the management of ST-elevation MI.

Question

Should patients presenting with NSTE-ACS receive DAPT?

Answer

Yes, DAPT with aspirin and either clopidogrel, prasugrel, or ticagrelor is recommended on admission for these patients.

CHAPTER 6

ACE INHIBITORS IN CONGESTIVE HEART FAILURE: THE CONSENSUS TRIAL

Anthony Carnicelli

Effects of Enalapril on Mortality in Severe Congestive Heart Failure. Results of the Cooperative North Scandinavian Enalapril Survival Study (CONSENSUS)

The CONSENSUS Trial Study Group. *N Engl J Med*. 1987;316(23):1429–1435

BACKGROUND

Prior to this study, therapy for patients with congestive heart failure (CHF) and reduced ejection fraction (EF) focused on symptom control using diuretics and contractility agents, and studies of afterload reduction with vasodilators such as nitrates and hydralazine had only shown nonsignificant trends toward mortality reduction. Although angiotensin-converting enzyme (ACE) inhibitors were thought to improve prognosis in this population and lead to hemodynamic and symptomatic improvement, their effects on mortality were unknown.

OBJECTIVES

To evaluate the effect of the ACE inhibitor enalapril on mortality among patients with severe CHF and reduced EF.

METHODS

Randomized, double-blind, placebo-controlled trial at 35 sites and 3 countries between 1985 and 1986.

Patients

253 patients. Inclusion criteria included CHF (defined as history of heart disease with symptoms of dyspnea and/or fatigue, signs of fluid retention, lack of primary pulmonary disease, and radiographically enlarged heart size) and New York Heart Association (NYHA) class IV symptoms. Exclusion criteria included hemodynamically significant aortic or mitral valve stenosis, myocardial infarction within 2 months prior, unstable angina, right heart failure due to pulmonary disease, or serum creatinine >3.39 mg/dL.

Interventions

Enalapril (2.5 mg twice daily for 1 week then 10 mg twice daily if tolerated) versus placebo. Additional dose increases were allowed based on clinical response up to a maximum dose of 20 mg twice daily. Additional vasodilators (nitrates, hydralazine, and/or prazosin) were permitted to treat worsening symptoms. All patients also received conventional CHF therapy.

Outcomes

The primary outcome was all-cause mortality at 6 months. Secondary outcomes included all-cause mortality at 12 months and during the study period.

KEY RESULTS

- All-cause mortality was lower in the enalapril group at 6 months (26% vs. 44%, RR 0.60, $p = 0.002$), 12 months (36% vs. 52%, RR 0.69, $p = 0.001$), and over the study period (39% vs. 54%, RR 0.73, $p = 0.003$).
- The reduction in mortality in the enalapril group was attributable to decreased death from the progression of heart failure (22% vs. 44%, $p = 0.001$).
- A greater proportion of patients in the enalapril group experienced improvement in NYHA functional class (42% vs. 22%, $p = 0.001$).

STUDY CONCLUSIONS

The addition of enalapril to conventional therapy in patients with severe CHF with reduced EF decreases mortality and improves symptoms. The beneficial effect on mortality is due to a reduction in death from the progression of heart failure.

COMMENTARY

CONSENSUS was the first trial to evaluate the effect of ACE inhibition on mortality and heart failure symptoms among patients with severe CHF with reduced EF. Caveats include the disproportionate number of men (70%) and a relatively short duration of follow-up (12 months). Subsequent studies with longer follow-up periods have confirmed the CONSENSUS findings and demonstrated benefit in patients with less severe CHF (NYHA classes II and III). Based on these results, the 2013 ACCF/AHA guideline for the management of heart failure recommends ACE inhibitors in patients with heart failure with reduced EF to reduce morbidity and mortality.

Question

Should patients with CHF with reduced EF be treated with ACE inhibitors?

Answer

Yes, when added to conventional therapy, ACE inhibitor therapy in these patients is associated with a reduction in mortality as well as symptom improvement.

CRT IN ADVANCED HEART FAILURE: THE COMPANION TRIAL

CHAPTER 7

Michael C. Honigberg

Cardiac-Resynchronization Therapy With or Without an Implantable Defibrillator in Advanced Chronic Heart Failure

Bristow MR, Saxon LA, Boehmer J, et al. *N Engl J Med*. 2004;350(21):2140–2150

BACKGROUND

Prior to this study, patients with cardiomyopathy and heart failure (HF) with reduced ejection fraction (EF) were known to be at increased risk for sudden cardiac death secondary to tachyarrhythmias. In those with ventricular dyssynchrony due to intraventricular conduction delay, cardiac-resynchronization therapy (CRT) had been shown to improve symptoms and left ventricular function, although the role of prophylactic CRT with or without an implantable cardioverter-defibrillator (ICD) in these populations remained unclear.

OBJECTIVES

To assess whether CRT with or without ICD improves outcomes in patients with advanced HF and intraventricular conduction delay compared to optimal medical therapy (OMT).

METHODS

Randomized, unblinded trial at 128 US hospitals between 2000 and 2002.

Patients

1,520 patients. Inclusion criteria included ischemic or nonischemic cardiomyopathy, New York Heart Association (NYHA) class III or IV HF with ≥1 HF admission in the last 12 months, left ventricular EF ≤35%, QRS duration ≥120 milliseconds and PR ≥150 milliseconds, sinus rhythm, and no other clinical indication for a pacemaker or defibrillator.

Interventions

CRT versus CRT with ICD versus no resynchronization therapy. All patients received OMT (diuretics, ACE inhibitors, beta blockers, and spironolactone).

Outcomes

The primary outcome was a composite of death or hospitalization from any cause. Secondary outcomes included all-cause death, death from or hospitalization for cardiovascular causes, and death from or hospitalization for HF.

KEY RESULTS

- The composite of death or hospitalization from any cause was lower in patients receiving CRT (56% vs. 68% in those receiving no resynchronization therapy, $p = 0.014$) and CRT with ICD (56% vs. 68% in those receiving no resynchronization therapy, $p = 0.01$).
- Death or hospitalization due to HF was also less frequent among patients receiving CRT (34% risk reduction, $p = 0.002$) or CRT with ICD (40% risk reduction, $p < 0.001$) compared to those not receiving resynchronization therapy.
- Treatment with CRT with ICD was associated with lower all-cause death (HR 0.64, 95% CI 0.48–0.86, $p = 0.003$) than patients receiving no resynchronization.

STUDY CONCLUSIONS

In patients with advanced HF and prolonged QRS interval, CRT decreases the risk of hospitalization or death and, when combined with ICD, reduces mortality.

COMMENTARY

Whereas preceding studies focused on symptoms and quality of life, COMPANION was the first to provide morbidity and mortality data to support CRT in patients with advanced HF. Based on this trial, the FDA approved combination CRT-ICD devices for patients with HF, reduced EF, and intraventricular conduction delay. The 2013 ACCF/AHA heart failure guidelines recommend CRT for patients with LVEF ≤35%, QRS duration ≥150 milliseconds, and NYHA class II–IV HF. The indications for ICD therapy for primary prevention of sudden cardiac death are similar to those for CRT, and the majority of CRT devices implanted today also possess ICD capability.

Question

Should patients with advanced HF and prolonged QRS receive CRT?

Answer

Yes, CRT decreases the risk of hospitalization or death and improves symptoms in this population, and the addition of an ICD decreases the risk of death.

CHAPTER 8

BETA BLOCKERS IN CHRONIC HEART FAILURE: THE COMET TRIAL

Michael C. Honigberg

Comparison of Carvedilol and Metoprolol on Clinical Outcomes in Patients With Chronic Heart Failure in the Carvedilol or Metoprolol European Trial (COMET): Randomised Controlled Trial

Poole-Wilson PA, Swedberg K, Cleland JG, et al. *Lancet*. 2003;362(9377):7–13

BACKGROUND
Despite the ability of beta blockers to improve symptoms and survival in chronic heart failure (HF), it was unclear if those effects were due to an overall "class effect" or particular pharmacologic properties such as specific blockade of β1-receptors versus nonselective blockade of β1-, β2-, and α1-adrenergic receptors. Prior to this study, β1-selective and nonselective beta blockers had not been directly compared with respect to HF outcomes.

OBJECTIVES
To compare the effects of carvedilol (nonselective beta blocker) and metoprolol (β1-selective beta blocker) on morbidity and mortality among patients with mild to severe chronic HF.

METHODS
Randomized, double-blind trial at 317 sites in 15 European countries between 1996 and 1999.

Patients
3,029 patients. Inclusion criteria included chronic symptomatic HF (New York Heart Association class II–IV) with reduced ejection fraction (≤35% or left ventricular end-diastolic diameter ≥6 cm with fractional shortening ≤20%), ≥1 cardiac admission in the prior 2 years, and a stable HF medication regimen including diuretics and ACE inhibitors. Exclusion criteria included recent acute coronary syndrome or stroke, poorly controlled hypertension or ventricular arrhythmia, and significant valvular disease.

Interventions
Carvedilol (3.125 mg twice daily, increased to target dose of 25 mg twice daily) versus metoprolol tartrate (5 mg twice daily, increased to target dose of 50 mg twice daily). Patients were followed for a mean of 58 months.

Outcomes
The primary outcomes were all-cause mortality and a composite of all-cause mortality and all-cause hospital admission. Secondary outcomes included cardiovascular mortality, noncardiovascular mortality, and sudden death.

KEY RESULTS

- Patients receiving carvedilol had lower all-cause mortality (34% vs. 40%; HR 0.83, 95% CI 0.74–0.93, $p = 0.002$), a finding that was driven by a reduction in cardiovascular death.
- There was no statistically significant difference in the composite outcome of death and all-cause admission (74% vs. 76%, $p = 0.122$).
- At 4-month follow-up, the carvedilol group had small but statistically significantly greater reductions in heart rate and SBP (–1.6 bpm and –1.8 mm Hg, respectively) compared to the metoprolol group.

CONCLUSIONS

Carvedilol reduces all-cause mortality compared with metoprolol tartrate in patients with chronic systolic HF.

COMMENTARY

COMET was done in part to assess whether carvedilol's properties (nonselective adrenergic blockade, insulin-sensitizing and antioxidant effects) confer an advantage compared to β1-selective agents like metoprolol and bisoprolol. Caveats include inequivalent metoprolol and carvedilol doses and potentially inadequate metoprolol dosing based on differential heart rate reductions; COMET also utilized short-acting rather than long-acting metoprolol formulation, the latter of which yielded survival benefit in other studies. As a result, the exact mechanisms underlying the study findings remain unclear, and the 2013 ACCF/AHA guidelines recommend bisoprolol, carvedilol, and metoprolol succinate as options in patients with chronic systolic HF.

Question

Is carvedilol a reasonable choice in the treatment of chronic HF with reduced ejection fraction?

Answer

Yes, although methodological limitations prevent definitive conclusions about its superiority over β1-selective beta blockers.

ANTIPLATELET THERAPY FOR PREVENTING VASCULAR EVENTS

Anubodh Varshney

Collaborative Overview of Randomised Trials of Antiplatelet Therapy – I: Prevention of Death, Myocardial Infarction, and Stroke by Prolonged Antiplatelet Therapy in Various Categories of Patients

Antiplatelet Trialists' Collaboration. *BMJ*. 1994;308(6921):81–106

BACKGROUND

By the early 1990s, there was evidence that antiplatelet therapy reduced vascular death and events in high-risk patients with acute or remote myocardial infarction (MI), stroke, or transient ischemic attack (TIA). However, the benefit and the risk/benefit balance in lower-risk patients, especially individuals with no history of these conditions, remained unknown. Data about the optimal agent, dose, and duration for antiplatelet therapy were also lacking.

OBJECTIVES

To assess the effects of antiplatelet therapy in more detail and breadth, in part by evaluating the effects of prolonged antiplatelet therapy on vascular events in patients of various risk categories.

METHODS

Meta-analysis of 174 randomized trials available for review by March 1990.

Patients

Approximately 110,000 patients, ranging from low-risk individuals (for whom the goal was primary prevention of vascular events) to those with varying degrees of higher risk. Four high-risk groups were defined: those with acute MI, prior MI, prior stroke/TIA, or other high-risk conditions.

Interventions

The meta-analysis evaluated 145 trials comparing antiplatelet therapy versus no antiplatelet therapy and 29 trials comparing one antiplatelet regimen versus another. Antiplatelet therapy was required for ≥1 month with agents whose primary mechanism was inhibition of platelet aggregation and/or adhesion.

Outcomes

The primary outcomes were vascular events (including nonfatal MI, nonfatal stroke, or vascular death) and nonvascular deaths.

KEY RESULTS

- Compared to those in the control group, high-risk patients receiving antiplatelet therapy – including those with acute MI (10% vs. 14%, $p < 0.001$), prior MI (13% vs. 17%, $p < 0.001$), prior stroke/TIA (18% vs. 22%, $p < 0.001$), or other high-risk conditions (7% vs. 9%, $p < 0.001$) – experienced lower vascular event rates without increases in nonvascular deaths.
- There were no statistically significant differences in vascular event rates among low-risk patients (4.5% vs. 4.8%, $p = 0.09$).
- There was no evidence that, compared to aspirin doses of 75 to 325 mg/day (the most frequently used regimens), higher doses or other antiplatelet agents were more effective at preventing vascular events.

STUDY CONCLUSIONS

Antiplatelet therapy, via either aspirin at doses of 75 to 325 mg/day or other regimens, is protective against MI, stroke, and death among high-risk patients. However, there was no clear evidence on the risk/benefit balance of antiplatelet therapy as primary prevention among low-risk patients.

COMMENTARY

By aggregating results from a large number of trials, this meta-analysis provided strong evidence that antiplatelet therapy – independent of specific regimen – is beneficial in high-risk patients in a range of settings. It also revealed that aspirin was beneficial as secondary prevention not only in patients with acute MI, prior MI, and prior TIA/stroke, but also those with a history of angina, bypass surgery, or angioplasty. Over 20 years later, aspirin remains codified in the 2011 AHA/ACCF guidelines for secondary prevention in patients with cardiovascular disease.

Question

Should patients at high risk for vascular events receive antiplatelet therapy?

Answer

Yes, in the absence of contraindications, prolonged antiplatelet therapy, either with aspirin or another agent, provides secondary prevention against vascular events in these patients.

CHAPTER 10

STATIN THERAPY AFTER ACS: PROVE IT-TIMI 22

Michael C. Honigberg

Intensive Versus Moderate Lipid Lowering With Statins After Acute Coronary Syndromes

Cannon CP, Braunwald E, McCabe CH, et al. *N Engl J Med.* 2004;350(15):1495–1504

BACKGROUND

Prior to this study, randomized studies had shown the cardiovascular benefits of statins. In turn, guidelines in the early 2000s recommended that patients with coronary artery disease (CAD) be treated with statins or other agents to a target low-density lipoprotein (LDL) level of <100 mg/dL. However, it was unknown whether further lowering LDL cholesterol in the setting of acute coronary syndromes (ACS) yielded additional reduction in cardiovascular risk.

OBJECTIVES

To compare clinical outcomes for high- and moderate-intensity statin therapy in patients recently hospitalized for ACS.

METHODS

Randomized controlled trial at 349 sites in 8 countries between 2000 and 2001.

Patients

4,162 patients hospitalized in stable condition for unstable angina, non–ST-elevation myocardial infarction (MI), or ST-elevation MI within the prior 10 days. Inclusion criteria included baseline total cholesterol <240 mg/dL or, if on long-term statin therapy, <200 mg/dL. Exclusion criteria included use of any statin at a dose of 80 mg daily, other CYP3A4-inhibiting medications, or nonstatin lipid-lowering therapy (e.g., niacin, fibrates) that could not be stopped before randomization.

Interventions

High-intensity treatment with atorvastatin (80 mg daily) versus moderate-intensity treatment with pravastatin (40 mg daily). Patients were followed for a mean of 2 years.

Outcomes

The primary outcome was a composite of all-cause mortality, unstable angina, MI, revascularization ≥30 days after randomization, and stroke. Secondary outcomes included components of the primary outcome, along with nonfatal MI and death from CAD.

KEY RESULTS

- At 2 years, the atorvastatin group had a lower rate of the primary outcome (22.4% vs. 26.3%, $p = 0.005$).
- Nearly all components of the primary outcome favored atorvastatin with the exception of stroke, which was rare and similar between the two groups.
- Atorvastatin was associated with a nonstatistically significant 28% reduction in all-cause mortality ($p = 0.07$).
- Patients in the atorvastatin group experienced greater LDL reduction, from a baseline of 106 mg/dL in both groups to a median LDL of 62 mg/dL, compared to a median LDL of 95 mg/dL in the pravastatin group.

STUDY CONCLUSIONS

Among patients with recent ACS, high-intensity statin therapy confers greater protection against death or major cardiovascular events than moderate-intensity therapy.

COMMENTARY

This study was pivotal for changing how statins are used to reduce cardiovascular risk. Not only did nearly all study outcomes favor high-intensity treatment, but the benefits were more rapid than those seen in earlier studies (days vs. months). Caveats include short follow-up duration and higher and unclear rates of study withdrawal (>30% in both groups at 2 years) compared to previous trials. On the basis of PROVE IT-TIMI 22 and subsequent trials, high-intensity statin therapy prior to discharge is now considered the standard of care for patients admitted with ACS regardless of baseline LDL.[1,2]

Question

Should patients with recent ACS receive high-intensity statin therapy for secondary prevention?

Answer

Yes, when initiated early, high-dose statin therapy can reduce cardiovascular morbidity and mortality compared to moderate-dose regimens.

References

1. American College of Emergency Physicians; Society for Cardiovascular Angiography and Interventions; O'Gara PT, Kushner FG, Ascheim DD, et al. 2013 ACCF/AHA guideline for the management of ST-elevation myocardial infarction: A report of the American College of Cardiology Foundation/American Heart Association Task Force on Practice Guidelines. *J Am Coll Cardiol.* 2013;61(4):e78–e140.
2. Amsterdam EA, Wenger NK, Brindis RG, et al; American College of Cardiology; American Heart Association Task Force on Practice Guidelines; Society for Cardiovascular Angiography and Interventions; Society of Thoracic Surgeons; American Association for Clinical Chemistry. 2014 AHA/ACC guideline for the management of patients with non-ST-elevation acute coronary syndromes: A report of the American College of Cardiology/American Heart Association Task Force on Practice Guidelines. *J Am Coll Cardiol.* 2014;64(24):e139–e228.

CHAPTER 11

TRANSCATHETER AORTIC VALVE IMPLANTATION: THE PARTNER B TRIAL

Anthony Carnicelli

Transcatheter Aortic-Valve Implantation for Aortic Stenosis in Patients Who Cannot Undergo Surgery

Leon MB, Smith CR, Mack M, et al. *N Engl J Med.* 2010;363(17):1597–1607

BACKGROUND

Although surgical valve replacement was known to reduce the high morbidity and mortality from aortic stenosis (AS), many AS patients were not surgical candidates due to high surgical risk from advanced age, left ventricular dysfunction, or multiple comorbidities. In these cases, less invasive treatments such as transcatheter aortic valve implantation (TAVI) were felt to be potentially beneficial.

OBJECTIVES

To compare mortality and hospitalization rates after TAVI with standard therapy.

METHODS

Randomized, open-label, comparative trial at 21 sites in 3 countries between 2007 and 2009.

Patients

358 patients. Inclusion criteria included severe AS (valve area <0.8 cm^2, valve index <0.5 cm^2/m^2, mean valve gradient ≥40 mm Hg, or peak velocity ≥4 m/sec), New York Heart Association class II–IV heart failure symptoms, and poor surgical candidacy (presence of coexisting conditions associated with ≥50% predicted postoperative 30-day risk of death or serious irreversible condition). Exclusion criteria included unicuspid, bicuspid, or noncalcified aortic valve, acute myocardial infarction, substantial coronary artery disease requiring revascularization, recent stroke or transient ischemic attack (TIA), severe aortic or mitral regurgitation, and left ventricular ejection fraction <20%.

Interventions

TAVI with a bovine pericardial valve versus standard therapy (primarily balloon aortic valvuloplasty).

Outcomes

The primary outcome was death from any cause. Secondary outcomes included death from cardiovascular cause, death from any cause or repeat hospitalization, death from any cause or major stroke, TIA or stroke, and any vascular complication.

KEY RESULTS

- At 1 year, the TAVI group had lower rates of death from any cause (30.7% vs. 49.7%, $p < 0.001$), cardiovascular cause (19.6% vs. 41.9%, $p < 0.001$), any cause or repeat hospitalization (42.5% vs. 70.4%, $p < 0.001$), and any cause or major stroke (33.0% vs. 50.3%, $p = 0.001$).
- TAVI was associated with higher rates of TIA or stroke (10.6% vs. 4.5%, $p = 0.04$) and vascular complications (32.4% vs. 7.3%, $p < 0.001$).

STUDY CONCLUSIONS

In patients with severe AS who were not suitable surgical candidates, TAVI reduced the rates of death from any cause but resulted in a higher incidence of major strokes and major vascular events when compared to standard therapy.

COMMENTARY

TAVI represents a major breakthrough in the treatment of AS. PARTNER B demonstrated that while standard therapy did not alter the natural history of severe AS for patients with prohibitive surgical risk, TAVI conferred marked benefits in terms of mortality and symptom improvement. Subsequent follow-up data revealed a persistent mortality reduction at 5 years.[1] However, the risk for vascular complications (number needed to harm = 4) and high incidence of stroke and TIA (number needed to harm = 16) – likely related to atheroembolism – should be considered. The incidence of paravalvular leak is also more common after TAVI than surgical valve replacement. Alternative deployment systems and cerebral protection devices have subsequently been developed to attempt to reduce the frequency of atheroembolic events.

Question

Should TAVI be considered as a therapeutic option for patients with severe AS who are poor surgical candidates?

Answer

Yes, in appropriately selected patients, TAVI can reduce the risk of death, but at the expense of increased risk of stroke and vascular complications.

References

1. Kapadia SR, Leon MB, Makkar RR, et al; PARTNER trial investigators. 5-year outcomes of transcatheter aortic valve replacement compared with standard treatment for patients with inoperable aortic stenosis (PARTNER 1): A randomised controlled trial. *Lancet.* 2015;385(9986):2485–2491.

CHAPTER 12

ANGIOPLASTY VERSUS t-PA IN MYOCARDIAL INFARCTION: THE PAMI-1 STUDY

Anubodh Varshney

A Comparison of Immediate Angioplasty With Thrombolytic Therapy for Acute Myocardial Infarction. The Primary Angioplasty in Myocardial Infarction Study Group. Grines CL, Browne KF, Marco J, et al. *N Engl J Med.* 1993;328(10):673–679

BACKGROUND

Systemic thrombolysis was the standard of care for acute ST-elevation myocardial infarction (STEMI) in the early 1990s, but its success was limited by recurrent myocardial ischemia, major bleeding, and failure to achieve arterial patency. Although percutaneous transluminal coronary angioplasty (PTCA) had demonstrated benefits as rescue therapy after failed thrombolysis, there were no large prospective evaluations of outcomes between immediate PTCA and thrombolysis.

OBJECTIVES

To compare clinical outcomes of immediate PTCA versus thrombolysis in patients with STEMI.

METHODS

Randomized controlled trial at 12 clinical centers in the United States and France between 1990 and 1992.

Patients

395 patients. Inclusion criteria included presentation within 12 hours of onset of ischemic chest pain with ≥1-mm ST-segment elevation in ≥2 contiguous electrocardiography leads. Exclusion criteria included complete left bundle branch block, cardiogenic shock, and high bleeding risk.

Interventions

Immediate PTCA (via diagnostic angiography and angioplasty of all lesions within the infarct-related vessel) versus thrombolysis (100 mg IV tissue plasminogen activator [t-PA] over 3 hours). All patients received medical therapy with oxygen, nitroglycerin, aspirin, and heparin. Patients randomized to PTCA were referred for coronary artery bypass graft surgery if left main, 3-vessel, or other high-risk disease was identified.

Outcomes

The primary outcome was the composite of mortality and reinfarction, measured during hospitalization and at 6 months follow-up. Secondary outcomes included intracranial bleeding, other bleeding, and arrhythmias.

KEY RESULTS

- The primary outcome was lower in the PTCA group in the hospital (5.1% vs. 12.0%, $p = 0.02$) and at 6 months (8.5% vs. 16.8%, $p = 0.02$)
- Hemorrhagic strokes occurred more commonly in the t-PA group (2.0% vs. 0.0%, $p = 0.05$) while ventricular fibrillation occurred more commonly in the PTCA group (6.7% vs. 2.0%, $p = 0.02$).
- There were no significant differences in left ventricular ejection fraction at 6 weeks.

STUDY CONCLUSIONS

Compared to thrombolysis with t-PA, immediate PTCA reduced the combined occurrence of death and nonfatal reinfarction, resulted in similar left ventricular systolic function, and led to a lower rate of intracranial hemorrhage among patients with STEMI.

COMMENTARY

Unlike earlier studies, PAMI-1 was large enough to evaluate differences in outcomes between immediate PTCA and thrombolysis. The study population was older and sicker than those in prior work, possibly contributing to higher rates of bleeding and death, especially in the t-PA arm. Given the favorable outcomes seen with immediate PTCA, this trial strengthened evidence for immediate angioplasty, particularly among those at high risk for vascular events. Furthermore, it helped build the foundation for timely percutaneous coronary intervention (PCI) as the current standard of care for STEMI patients presenting to PCI-capable centers.[1]

Question

Is immediate PCI a preferable strategy to t-PA among patients with STEMI?

Answer

Yes, although consideration should also be given to local settings and resources (e.g., availability of, and time required to obtain, PCI).

References

1. American College of Emergency Physicians; Society for Cardiovascular Angiography and Interventions; O'Gara PT, Kushner FG, Ascheim DD, et al. 2013 ACCF/AHA guideline for the management of ST-elevation myocardial infarction: A report of the American College of Cardiology Foundation/American Heart Association Task Force on Practice Guidelines. *J Am Coll Cardiol.* 2013;61(4):e78–e140.

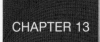

ASPIRIN AND THROMBOLYSIS IN MYOCARDIAL INFARCTION: THE ISIS-2 TRIAL

CHAPTER 13

Anubodh Varshney

Randomised Trial of Intravenous Streptokinase, Oral Aspirin, Both, or Neither Among 17,187 Cases of Suspected Acute Myocardial Infarction: ISIS-2

ISIS-2 (Second International Study of Infarct Survival) Collaborative Group. *Lancet.* 1988;2(8607):349–360

BACKGROUND
Prior to this study, small trials had indicated that early fibrinolysis with streptokinase and platelet inhibition with aspirin could reduce cardiovascular morbidity and mortality in patients with acute myocardial infarction (MI). However, the post-MI "time window" during which streptokinase provided benefit, and the potential for aspirin to mitigate the risk of reocclusion after fibrinolysis, remained unknown.

OBJECTIVES
To evaluate the effects of intravenous streptokinase and oral aspirin on mortality in patients presenting with acute MI.

METHODS
Randomized, placebo-controlled trial with 2 × 2 factorial design at 417 hospitals in 16 countries from 1985 to 1987.

Patients
17,187 patients. Inclusion criteria included presentation ≤24 hours of symptoms of suspected MI and no contraindication to streptokinase or aspirin (e.g., history of either stroke, gastrointestinal hemorrhage, or ulcer). Exclusion criteria included recent trauma or arterial puncture, and severe hypertension.

Interventions
Intravenous streptokinase (1-hour infusion of 1.5 MU) versus oral enteric-coated aspirin (160 mg/day for 1 month) versus both treatments versus neither.

Outcomes
The primary outcome was vascular mortality. Secondary outcomes included all-cause mortality, in-hospital adverse events (e.g., bleeding), stroke, and reinfarction.

KEY RESULTS
- Compared to placebo, vascular mortality was lower in the aspirin (9.4% vs. 11.8%, RR 0.80, $p < 0.001$) and streptokinase (9.2% vs. 12.0%, RR 0.77, $p < 0.001$) groups.
- Receipt of both aspirin and streptokinase led to lower vascular mortality (8.0% vs. 13.2% in placebo group, $p < 0.001$).

- The benefit of streptokinase persisted up to 24 hours from symptom onset but was greatest in patients who received it in the 0 to 4-hour time window; time of administration did not affect benefit in the aspirin group.
- Compared to placebo, patients receiving streptokinase had higher rates of bleeding requiring transfusion (0.5% vs. 0.2%, $p < 0.001$) and cerebral hemorrhage (0.1% vs. 0.0%, $p < 0.02$), but not total strokes (0.7% vs. 0.8%, $p > 0.05$).

STUDY CONCLUSIONS

In patients presenting with acute MI, streptokinase and aspirin confer independent and additive vascular mortality benefit compared to placebo.

COMMENTARY

ISIS-2 was important as the first trial to demonstrate the clinical efficacy of aspirin as an antiplatelet agent in reducing vascular mortality in acute MI. Caveats include randomization related to thrombolytics despite existing evidence of their benefit from preceding studies and an apparent lack of clinical equipoise. Results from ISIS-2 helped spur adoption of antiplatelet therapy in the treatment of acute MI and expanded the use of fibrinolytics to those presenting more than 4 hours after pain onset. Nearly 30 years later, these results still inform clinical guidelines, which recommend aspirin in ACS and, in the case of ST-elevation MI, thrombolysis in the absence of timely access to percutaneous coronary intervention.[1,2]

Question

Should aspirin and thrombolysis be considered in patients presenting less than 24 hours after ACS onset?

Answer

Yes, aspirin reduces mortality in ACS and thrombolysis should be considered for ST-elevation MI when timely percutaneous coronary intervention is unavailable.

References

1. Amsterdam EA, Wenger NK, Brindis RG, et al; American College of Cardiology; American Heart Association Task Force on Practice Guidelines; Society for Cardiovascular Angiography and Interventions; Society of Thoracic Surgeons; American Association for Clinical Chemistry. 2014 AHA/ACC guideline for the management of patients with non-ST-elevation acute coronary syndromes: A report of the American College of Cardiology/American Heart Association Task Force on Practice Guidelines. *J Am Coll Cardiol.* 2014;64(24):e139–e228.
2. O'Gara PT, Kushner FG, Ascheim DD, et al; American College of Emergency Physicians; Society for Cardiovascular Angiography and Interventions. 2013 ACCF/AHA guideline for the management of ST-elevation myocardial infarction: A report of the American College of Cardiology Foundation/American Heart Association Task Force on Practice Guidelines. *J Am Coll Cardiol.* 2013;61(4):e78–e140.

CHAPTER 14

HEPARIN IN ACS WITHOUT ST ELEVATION

Elizabeth A. Richey

Unfractionated Heparin and Low-Molecular-Weight Heparin in Acute Coronary Syndrome Without ST Elevation: A Meta-Analysis

Eikelboom JW, Anand SS, Malmberg K, Weitz JI, Ginsberg JS, Yusuf S. *Lancet.* 2000;355(9219):1936–1942

BACKGROUND

Prior to this analysis, anticoagulation with unfractionated heparin (UFH) or low–molecular-weight heparin (LMWH) was commonly used in the treatment of acute coronary syndrome (ACS) without ST elevation. However, conflicting evidence and opinions remained, both about the additional benefit of anticoagulation using heparin over treatment with aspirin alone, as well as the optimal heparin agent and treatment duration.

OBJECTIVES

To evaluate and compare the effect of UFH and LMWH on death, myocardial infarction (MI), and major bleeding among patients with ACS without ST elevation.

METHODS

A meta-analysis of 12 randomized trials published between 1988 and 1999.

Patients

17,157 patients with ACS without ST elevation treated with aspirin. Study inclusion in the meta-analysis required randomization, evaluation of patients with unstable angina or non–Q-wave MI, and aspirin treatment among all study participants.

Interventions

The meta-analysis involved three comparisons: UFH versus placebo or untreated controls, LMWH versus placebo or untreated controls, and UFH versus LMWH.

Outcomes

The primary outcome was a composite of death or MI. Major bleeding was the primary safety outcome. Secondary outcomes were recurrent angina and need for revascularization.

KEY RESULTS

- In pooled analysis of the 8 studies comparing either UFH or LMWH with placebo or untreated controls, the rate of death or MI was lower among patients receiving UFH or LMWH (4.5% vs. 7.4%, OR 0.53, 95% CI 0.38–0.73, $p < 0.001$).
- Among the 5 trials that directly compared LMWH with UFH, patients treated with LMWH had a 2.2% rate of death or MI compared to 2.3% among those receiving UFH (OR 0.88, 95% CI 0.69–1.12, $p = 0.34$).

- There was no difference in risk of major bleeding among patients treated with LMWH versus UFH (OR 1.00, 95% CI 0.64–1.57, $p = 0.99$).
- In trials of longer-term anticoagulation (up to 3 months), LMWH was associated with an increased risk of major bleeding (OR 2.26, 95% CI 1.63–3.14, $p < 0.001$) and no reduction in death or MI compared to placebo.

STUDY CONCLUSIONS

Short-term UFH or LMWH halves the risk of MI or death in aspirin-treated patients with ACS without ST elevation. There is no convincing difference in efficacy or safety between the two agents or data to support the long-term use of LMWH beyond the first 7 days.

COMMENTARY

This meta-analysis helped define management of aspirin-treated patients with non–ST-elevation MI and unstable angina. Notably, a reduction in nonfatal MI was the primary driver of observed results, including in studies done prior to widespread use of $P2Y_{12}$ inhibitors. Subsequently, prospective evaluations of patients undergoing early invasive treatment revealed that UFH and LMWH have comparable efficacy among those receiving contemporary dual antiplatelet therapy, with modestly increased bleeding from LMWH. Collectively, these studies have informed the 2014 AHA/ACC guidelines for management of ACS without ST elevation, which recommend anticoagulation with either LMWH (class A recommendation) or UFH (class B) as part of both conservative and early invasive treatment strategies.

Question

Should patients presenting with ACS without ST elevation receive short-term heparin therapy?

Answer

Yes, LMWH or UFH is beneficial among these patients as part of both conservative and early invasive treatment strategies.

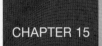

CHAPTER 15

PCI VERSUS CABG FOR SEVERE CAD: THE SYNTAX TRIAL

Michael C. Honigberg

Percutaneous Coronary Intervention Versus Coronary-Artery Bypass Grafting for Severe Coronary Artery Disease

Serruys PW, Morice MC, Kappetein AP, et al. *N Engl J Med.* 2009;360(10):961–972

BACKGROUND

Before the availability of drug-eluting stents, studies had suggested that coronary artery bypass graft (CABG) led to superior outcomes in symptomatic coronary artery disease (CAD) compared to percutaneous coronary intervention (PCI) with balloon angioplasty or bare-metal stents. However, the comparative effects of CABG and PCI in the era of drug-eluting stents were unclear. Few studies evaluating CABG and PCI had included patients with severe disease (i.e., left main or 3-vessel CAD) for whom existing guideline recommendations were to undergo CABG. Even fewer studies had compared outcomes using drug-eluting stents.

OBJECTIVES

To determine the optimal revascularization strategy for patients with untreated left main or 3-vessel CAD when both surgical and percutaneous options are feasible.

METHODS

Randomized controlled trial at 85 sites in the United States and 17 European countries between 2005 and 2007.

Patients

1,800 patients with previously untreated left main and 3-vessel CAD. Exclusion criteria included previous intervention, acute myocardial infarction (MI), need for concomitant surgery, and eligibility for either CABG or PCI but not both.

Interventions

PCI with drug-eluting stents versus CABG. Patients were followed for 12 months after intervention.

Outcomes

The primary outcome was a composite of death from any cause, stroke, MI, or repeat revascularization. Secondary outcomes included individual components of the primary outcome as well as death from cardiac and cardiovascular causes.

KEY RESULTS

- At 12 months, the composite primary outcome occurred more frequently in patients receiving PCI (17.8% vs. 12.4%, $p = 0.002$), a finding that appeared to be driven by a higher rate of repeat revascularization (13.5% vs. 5.9%, $p < 0.001$).
- Complete revascularization was achieved in a larger proportion of patients in the CABG group (63.2% vs. 56.7%, $p = 0.005$).
- The rate of stroke was higher in patients undergoing CABG (2.2% vs. 0.6%, $p = 0.003$).

STUDY CONCLUSIONS

CABG remains the standard of care for patients with left main or 3-vessel CAD given lower rates of the combined endpoint of major adverse cardiac or cerebrovascular events at 1 year.

COMMENTARY

SYNTAX was pivotal for reinforcing CABG as the standard of care for patients with severe CAD, a conclusion that was further underscored in follow-up studies at 3 and 5 years. Findings should be interpreted in view of the low percentage of women enrolled (22%), suboptimal medical therapy in the CABG group, and unclear reasons (e.g., differences in medical therapy or procedural complications) for higher than expected stroke rates in both groups. Additionally, post hoc analyses found that outcomes correlated with participants' SYNTAX scores (a disease severity score based on the location, severity, and extent of CAD determined at the time of catheterization) and that PCI and CABG were comparable among patients with lower SYNTAX scores.

Question

When both CABG and PCI are feasible, should most patients with left main or 3-vessel CAD undergo revascularization with CABG?

Answer

Yes, CABG is the preferred revascularization strategy in many of these situations, but the extent of CAD can also affect decisions regarding the optimal approach.

CHAPTER 16

ANTIARRHYTHMICS AND ICDs IN CHF: THE SCD-HeFT TRIAL

Anthony Carnicelli

Amiodarone or an Implantable Cardioverter-Defibrillator for Congestive Heart Failure
Bardy GH, Lee KL, Mark DB, et al. *N Engl J Med*. 2005;352(3):225–237

BACKGROUND

Prior to this study, congestive heart failure (CHF) with reduced ejection fraction (EF) was a known major risk factor for sudden cardiac death from ventricular arrhythmia. Medical therapy with the antiarrhythmic drug amiodarone and immediate cardioversion with an implantable cardioverter-defibrillator (ICD) were both theorized to prevent arrhythmias and reduce mortality.

OBJECTIVES

To evaluate whether amiodarone or ICD would decrease mortality in patients with mild-to-moderate CHF with reduced EF.

METHODS

Randomized, double-blind, placebo-controlled trial between 1997 and 2001. Blinding was used between amiodarone and placebo groups but no implanted sham device was used for comparison to the ICD group.

Patients

2,521 patients. Inclusion criteria included New York Heart Association (NYHA) class II or III CHF due to ischemic or nonischemic causes, and left ventricular EF ≤35%. Exclusion criteria included history of ventricular tachycardia or ventricular fibrillation, indication for pacemaker implantation, and reversible cardiomyopathy. Prespecified subgroups were based on CHF cause (ischemic vs. nonischemic) and NYHA class (II vs. III).

Interventions

Amiodarone (loading followed by weight-based daily maintenance doses) versus single-lead ICD (conservatively programmed, shock only) versus placebo. All groups received conventional heart failure therapy.

Outcomes

The primary outcome was death from any cause.

KEY RESULTS

- Compared to placebo, ICD therapy was associated with a lower risk of death (HR 0.77, 97.5% CI 0.62–0.96, p = 0.007); amiodarone was associated with a similar risk of death compared to placebo (HR 1.06, 97.5% CI 0.86–1.30, p = 0.53).
- Compared to placebo, ICD therapy was associated with a lower risk of death among patients with NYHA class II disease (HR 0.54, 97.5% CI 0.40–0.74, p < 0.001) but not in patients with class III disease (HR 1.16, 97.5% CI 0.84–1.61, p = 0.30).
- Amiodarone was associated with a similar risk of death compared to placebo among patients with NYHA class II disease (HR 0.85, 97.5% CI 0.65–1.11, p = 0.17) but a higher risk of death among patients with class III disease (HR 1.44, 97.5% CI 1.05–1.97, p = 0.01).

STUDY CONCLUSIONS

In patients with NYHA class II or III CHF and left ventricular EF ≤ 35%, amiodarone confers no mortality benefit. Single-lead, shock-only ICD therapy reduces overall mortality in patients with NYHA class II disease.

COMMENTARY

In addition to clarifying the effects of amiodarone in patients with mild-to-moderate CHF, SCD-HeFT demonstrated that ICD therapy could reduce mortality even in those without a prior history of cardiac arrest. Caveats include the need to consider the cost and complication risks associated with ICD implantation and maintenance, although these concerns may be mitigated by savings from the use of single-lead ICD and simplified follow-up schedules. The SCD-HeFT findings – most notably the absolute 7.2% 5-year mortality reduction, with a number needed to treat of 14 – informed the 2013 ACCF/AHA guideline for management of heart failure, which recommends ICD therapy for primary prevention in patients with CHF and LVEF ≤35% from ischemic or nonischemic causes and expected survival >1 year, at least 40 days postmyocardial infarction.

Question

Should patients with mild-to-moderate heart failure and LVEF ≤35% undergo ICD implantation for primary prevention of sudden cardiac death?

Answer

Yes, though consideration should also be given to an individual patient's risk for complications and expected survival.

CHAPTER 17

ACE INHIBITORS IN LV DYSFUNCTION: THE SAVE TRIAL

Anish Mehta

Effect of Captopril on Mortality and Morbidity in Patients With Left Ventricular Dysfunction After Myocardial Infarction. Results of the Survival and Ventricular Enlargement Trial. The SAVE Investigators.

Pfeffer MA, Braunwald E, Moyé LA, et al. *N Engl J Med*. 1992;327(10):669–677

BACKGROUND

Prior to this study, animal models had shown that angiotensin-converting enzyme (ACE) inhibitors could attenuate left ventricular (LV) dysfunction and improve survival after myocardial infarction (MI). While subsequent human studies confirmed the ability of ACE inhibition to attenuate ventricular dysfunction after MI, they were too small to assess its influence on survival.

OBJECTIVES

To determine whether long-term administration of captopril can reduce morbidity and mortality in patients with LV dysfunction after MI.

METHODS

Randomized, placebo-controlled, double-blind trial at 112 hospitals in the United States and Canada from 1987 to 1992.

Patients

2,231 adult patients post-MI. Inclusion criteria included ejection fraction (EF) ≤40%. Exclusion criteria included age ≥80 years, symptomatic HF, use of ACE inhibitor for hypertension, serum creatinine >2.5 mg/dL, and unstable course after MI.

Interventions

Captopril (25 mg 3 times daily at hospital discharge, titrated to 50 mg 3 times daily) versus placebo.

Outcomes

The primary outcome was all-cause mortality. Other outcomes included cardiovascular (CV) mortality, symptomatic HF requiring hospitalization, recurrent MI, and HF requiring open-label ACE inhibitors.

KEY RESULTS

- All-cause mortality was lower in the captopril group (20% vs. 25%, $p = 0.019$).
- CV mortality was lower in the captopril group (21% vs. 17%, $p = 0.014$).
- Fewer patients receiving captopril experienced hospitalization due to HF (14% vs. 17%, $p = 0.019$) or recurrent MI (12% vs. 15%, $p = 0.019$).
- The composite of CV death, HF requiring hospitalization, HF requiring ACE inhibitors, or recurrent MI occurred less frequently in the captopril group (32% vs. 40%, $p < 0.001$).

STUDY CONCLUSIONS

Long-term treatment with captopril in survivors of MI with asymptomatic LV dysfunction led to reduced mortality and CV morbidity.

COMMENTARY

SAVE was the first trial to show that ACE inhibitors improve survival in patients with LV dysfunction post-MI. Subsequent studies have expanded the indications for ACE inhibitors post-MI, with a meta-analysis suggesting that the greatest benefit accrues for those with high-risk features (e.g., EF ≤40%, anterior MI, and HF).[1] SAVE and subsequent work has informed the ACCF/AHA 2013 ST-elevation MI and 2014 non–ST-elevation acute coronary syndrome guidelines, both of which strongly recommend ACE inhibitors in patients with decreased EF after MI.

Question

Should patients with asymptomatic LV dysfunction after acute MI be treated with an ACE inhibitor?

Answer

Yes, ACE inhibitors reduce mortality and CV morbidity in these patients.

References

1. ACE Inhibitor Myocardial Infarction Collaborative Group. Indications for ACE inhibitors in the early treatment of acute myocardial infarction: Systematic overview of individual data from 100,000 patients in randomized trials. *Circulation.* 1998;97(22):2202–2212.

CHAPTER 18

DABIGATRAN FOR ATRIAL FIBRILLATION: THE RE-LY TRIAL

Zahir Kanjee ■ Joshua M. Liao

Dabigatran Versus Warfarin in Patients With Atrial Fibrillation

Connolly SJ, Ezekowitz MD, Yusuf S, et al. *N Engl J Med*. 2009;361(12):1139–1151

BACKGROUND

Although vitamin K antagonists (VKAs) have been traditionally used to prevent stroke in atrial fibrillation (AF), they are limited by significant dietary restrictions, drug interactions, and need for frequent laboratory monitoring. Prior to this study, however, efforts to replace VKAs with less burdensome medications were either ineffective or associated with increased bleeding risk or significant toxicity. Dabigatran etexilate is an oral direct thrombin inhibitor that showed encouraging results in preliminary studies.

OBJECTIVES

To assess whether dabigatran is noninferior to warfarin in preventing stroke or systemic embolism in patients with AF.

METHODS

Randomized, open-label controlled trial at 951 centers in 44 countries between 2005 and 2007.

Patients

18,113 patients with AF. Inclusion criteria included age ≥75 years (or 65 to 74 years with diabetes, hypertension, or coronary artery disease) and ≥1 of the following: previous stroke or transient ischemic attack (TIA), left ventricular ejection fraction <40%, heart failure with at least New York Heart Association class II symptoms within 6 months. Exclusion criteria included severe valvular disease, stroke within 14 days or severe stroke within 6 months, increased bleeding risk, creatinine clearance <30 mL/min, and active liver disease.

Interventions

Lower-dose dabigatran etexilate (110 mg twice daily) versus higher-dose dabigatran etexilate (150 mg twice daily) versus warfarin (goal INR 2.0 to 3.0).

Outcomes

The primary outcome was stroke or systemic embolism. The primary safety outcome was major hemorrhage. Other outcomes included stroke, systemic embolism, and death.

KEY RESULTS

- The annual rate of stroke or systemic embolism was 1.69% in the warfarin group compared to 1.53% in the lower-dose (RR 0.91, CI 0.74–1.11, $p < 0.001$ for non-inferiority) and 1.11% in the higher-dose (RR 0.66, CI 0.53–0.82, $p < 0.001$ for superiority) dabigatran groups.
- Compared to those in the warfarin group, annual rates of major bleeding were lower in the lower-dose dabigatran group (2.71% vs. 3.36%, $p = 0.003$); there was no statistically significant difference in rates between the higher-dose dabigatran and warfarin groups (3.11% vs. 3.36%, $p = 0.31$).
- Annual mortality rates were 4.13% in the warfarin group, compared to 3.75% in the lower-dose ($p = 0.13$) and 3.64% in higher-dose ($p = 0.051$) dabigatran groups.

STUDY CONCLUSIONS

Compared to warfarin, dabigatran at a dose of 110 mg was noninferior to warfarin in preventing stroke or systemic embolism and associated with less major hemorrhage among patients with AF. At a dose of 150 mg, dabigatran was superior to warfarin in preventing stroke or systemic embolism and associated with a similar rate of major bleeding.

COMMENTARY

RE-LY signaled a new era in anticoagulation. It was the first study to show that a direct oral anticoagulant (DOAC) could be a safe and effective alternative to VKAs, a finding followed soon afterward by similar investigations in AF of rivaroxaban, apixaban, and edoxaban. DOACs are now widely prescribed for stroke prevention in nonvalvular AF and are recommended, along with warfarin, as excellent options in the 2014 AHA/ACC AF guidelines.

Question

Are DOACs a safe and effective alternative to warfarin in patients with nonvalvular AF?

Answer

Yes, several agents offer comparable to improved outcomes with similar to improved rates of major bleeding.

CHAPTER 19

SPIRONOLACTONE IN SEVERE HF: THE RALES TRIAL

Mounica Vallurupalli

The effect of spironolactone on morbidity and mortality in patients with severe heart failure.

Pitt B, Zannad F, Remme WJ, et al. *N Engl J Med*. 1999;341(10):709–717

BACKGROUND

Prior to 1999, angiotensin-converting enzyme (ACE) inhibitors were the treatment of choice to suppress the formation of aldosterone in heart failure (HF). However, ACE inhibitors only transiently reduce aldosterone levels and small observational trials showed that further suppression of aldosterone could be beneficial. Direct aldosterone receptor blockers were not commonly used as adjunctive treatment given concerns of hyperkalemia and renal dysfunction.

OBJECTIVES

To assess the effect of the direct aldosterone receptor blocker spironolactone, in conjunction with standard therapy, on mortality in severe symptomatic systolic HF.

METHODS

Randomized, placebo-controlled, double-blind trial in 195 centers in 15 countries from 1995 to 1998.

Patients

1,663 patients. Inclusion criteria included New York Heart Association (NYHA) class IV HF within the past 6 months, NYHA class III or IV within 6 weeks of enrollment, treatment with an ACE inhibitor and loop diuretic, and left ventricular ejection fraction (EF) <35%. Exclusion criteria included primary operable valve disease, congenital heart disease, unstable angina, serum creatinine >2.5 mg/dL, serum potassium >5 mEq/L, or other life-threatening illness.

Interventions

Spironolactone (25 mg daily, titrated up to 50 mg daily for worsening HF or down for hyperkalemia) versus placebo. All patients received standard HF therapy, which included ACE inhibitors. Mean follow-up was 24 months.

Outcomes

The primary outcome was all-cause mortality. Secondary outcomes included death from cardiac causes, hospitalization for cardiac causes, combined incidence of death or hospitalization from cardiac causes, and change in NYHA class.

KEY RESULTS

- All-cause mortality was lower in the spironolactone group (35% vs. 46%, RR 0.70, 95% CI 0.60–0.82, $p < 0.001$).
- The spironolactone group also had lower rates of death from cardiac causes (27% vs. 37%, RR 0.69, 95% CI 0.58–0.82, $p < 0.001$) and hospitalization for cardiac causes (RR 0.70, 95% CI 0.59–0.82, $p < 0.001$).
- There were no statistically significant differences in serious hyperkalemia between the 2 groups (2% vs. 1%, $p = 0.42$).
- Gynecomastia and breast pain were more common in the spironolactone group ($p < 0.001$).

STUDY CONCLUSIONS

The addition of spironolactone to standard therapy reduces morbidity and mortality among patients with symptomatic severe systolic HF.

COMMENTARY

RALES definitively demonstrated that among patients with severe systolic HF, spironolactone could reduce morbidity and mortality when used concomitantly with ACE inhibitors without major adverse effects on renal function or serum potassium. In fact, the study was terminated early given the significant benefit observed in the spironolactone group. An important limitation is that only 10% of subjects received beta blockers, which were not yet standard of care at the time. Although not observed in RALES, spironolactone is also commonly associated with hyperkalemia in clinical practice. Based on the results from RALES and a subsequent study demonstrating similar benefits in patients with less severe HF, the 2013 ACCF/AHA HF guidelines strongly recommend aldosterone receptor antagonists for patients with EF <35% and NYHA class II–IV disease.

Question

Should patients with severe symptomatic systolic HF receive aldosterone receptor blockade in addition to ACE inhibitors?

Answer

Yes, barring significant renal dysfunction and baseline hyperkalemia, aldosterone receptor blockade reduces HF symptoms and all-cause mortality.

| CHAPTER 20 | CHOLESTEROL LOWERING IN CORONARY ARTERY DISEASE: THE 4S TRIAL |

Anthony Carnicelli

Randomized trial of cholesterol lowering in 4444 patients with coronary heart disease: The Scandinavian Simvastatin Survival Study (4S)

Scandinavian Simvastatin Survival Study Group. *Lancet.* 1994;344(8934):1383–1389

BACKGROUND

In the years preceding this study, hyperlipidemia was recognized as a major risk factor for coronary artery disease (CAD) and its sequelae. Although prior studies showed that cholesterol-lowering agents such as bile acid sequestrants and fibrates could lead to favorable reductions in CAD incidence and composite endpoints, none had demonstrated an effect on mortality. Without prospective evidence of mortality benefit, guidelines recommending cholesterol-lowering agents were greatly debated.

OBJECTIVES

To evaluate the effect of cholesterol lowering with simvastatin on morbidity and mortality in patients with CAD.

METHODS

Randomized, placebo-controlled trial at 94 sites in Scandinavia between 1988 and 1989.

Patients

4,444 patients. Inclusion criteria included age 35 to 70 years, CAD (defined as angina pectoris or myocardial infarction [MI] >6 months prior to randomization). Exclusion criteria included total cholesterol <212 or >309 mg/dL, triglycerides >221 mg/dL, unstable angina or MI within prior 6 months, hemodynamically significant valvular heart disease, stroke, and liver disease.

Interventions

Simvastatin (20 mg daily) versus placebo. At follow-up, dose adjustment up to 50 mg daily or down to 10 mg daily was allowed if necessary to achieve total cholesterol of 115 to 200 mg/dL.

Outcomes

The primary outcome was all-cause mortality. The secondary outcome was major coronary events (including coronary death, nonfatal acute MI, resuscitated cardiac arrest, and silent MI verified by electrocardiography). Additional outcomes included any coronary event and death or any atherosclerotic event.

KEY RESULTS

- All-cause mortality was lower in the simvastatin group (8.2% vs. 11.5%, RR 0.70, 95% CI 0.58–0.85, $p < 0.001$).
- Patients receiving simvastatin experienced lower rates of major coronary events (22.6% vs. 15.9%, RR 0.66, 95% CI 0.59–0.75, $p < 0.001$).
- The frequency of adverse events was similar in the 2 groups.

STUDY CONCLUSIONS

Long-term treatment with simvastatin is safe and improves survival in patients with CAD.

COMMENTARY

This study represented a major landmark in secondary prevention for cardiovascular disease. While other lipid-lowering agents had only shown modest reductions in cardiovascular outcomes, 4S was the first to show that cholesterol lowering with statin therapy confers a mortality benefit (number needed to treat = 30). In fact, the absolute risk reduction of 3.3% in the statin group was so significant that 4S was stopped early. Statin therapy also led to reductions in LDL (38% decrease) and total cholesterol (28% decrease), and a post hoc analysis found the additional benefit of reduced incidence of cerebrovascular events. Caveats include the disproportionate number of men (82%) and the low rate of aspirin use among participants (37%). Results from the 4S trial have contributed to the 2013 ACC/AHA cholesterol-treatment guidelines, which recommend statin use in patients with clinical atherosclerotic cardiovascular disease.

Question

Do patients with CAD benefit from statin therapy?

Answer

Yes, statins lead to improved morbidity and mortality in patients with CAD.

CRITICAL CARE

CHAPTER 21

GLUCOSE CONTROL IN ICU PATIENTS: THE NICE-SUGAR TRIAL

Melissa G. Lechner

Intensive Versus Conventional Glucose Control in Critically Ill Patients

Finfer S, Chittock DR, Su SY, et al. *N Engl J Med*. 2009;360(13):1283–1297

BACKGROUND

Prior to this study, hyperglycemia was recognized as a common condition associated with a wide range of adverse outcomes, including in critically ill patients. Based on retrospective analyses and small prospective randomized trials, professional organizations began widely encouraging tight glycemic control for patients in the intensive care unit (ICU). However, the mortality benefit reported in some studies was offset by high rates of hypoglycemia, and expert opinion and conclusions from meta-analyses remained split on the optimal intensity of glucose control in ICU patients.

OBJECTIVES

To determine whether intensive glucose control in ICU patients reduces mortality.

METHODS

Randomized controlled trial at 42 academic and community centers in Australia, New Zealand, and North America between 2004 and 2008. Randomization was stratified by admission type (operative or nonoperative).

Patients

6,104 ICU patients. Inclusion criteria included expected ICU stay ≥3 days. Exclusion criteria included age <18 years, admission for diabetic ketoacidosis or hyperosmolar state, and previous hypoglycemia without full neurologic recovery.

Interventions

Intensive glucose control (with blood glucose titrated to a goal of 81 to 108 mg/dL using intravenous insulin and routine glucose measurements) versus conventional glucose control (with a target of ≤180 mg/dL and discontinuation of insulin for blood glucose <144 mg/dL). Glucose levels were managed by clinical staff with guidance provided by a study treatment algorithm.

Outcomes

The primary outcome was death from any cause at 90 days. Secondary outcomes included survival time, cause-specific death, durations of mechanical ventilation, renal replacement therapy, and ICU and hospital stays. Serious hypoglycemia (blood glucose <40 mg/dL) was assessed.

KEY RESULTS

- Patients in the intensive glucose control group had higher 90-day mortality rates (27.5% vs. 24.9%; OR 1.14, 95% CI 1.02–1.28, $p = 0.02$) and higher rates of severe hypoglycemia (6.8% vs. 0.5%, $p < 0.001$).
- There were no statistically significant differences in the treatment effect within predefined subgroup pairs (nonoperative vs. operative patients, diabetics vs. non-diabetics, those with severe sepsis vs. without severe sepsis, Acute Physiology and Chronic Health Evaluation II score <25 vs. ≥25) with respect to 90-day mortality.
- There were no statistically significant differences between treatment groups in median ICU or hospital length of stay, or median days of mechanical ventilation or renal replacement therapy.

STUDY CONCLUSIONS

Intensive glucose control with a glucose target of 81 to 108 mg/dL increased mortality among adult ICU patients compared to conventional control, defined as a target <180 mg/dL.

COMMENTARY

This large, multinational trial established that tight glucose control was associated with more frequent severe hypoglycemia and increased overall mortality across all patient subgroups. Of note, NICE-SUGAR did not examine specific causes of mortality relevant to ICU patients or factors such as large glucose fluctuations or adequacy of caloric intake. Insulin was also administered by intravenous drip and discontinued after patients resumed eating or left the ICU, limiting generalizability to other hospital populations. The 2012 Society of Critical Care Medicine guidelines incorporate these findings and recommend controlling glucose <180 mg/dL and avoiding hypoglycemia in critically ill patients.

Question

Should critically ill patients receive intensive insulin control?

Answer

No, intensive control in critically ill patients increases mortality and produces more frequent severe hypoglycemia without improving other clinical outcomes.

CHAPTER 22

THERAPEUTIC HYPOTHERMIA AFTER CARDIAC ARREST: THE HACA TRIAL

Vivek T. Kulkarni

Mild Therapeutic Hypothermia to Improve the Neurologic Outcome After Cardiac Arrest
The Hypothermia After Cardiac Arrest Study Group. *N Engl J Med*. 2002;346(8):549–556

BACKGROUND
Historically, survivors of cardiac arrest (CA) have had poor neurologic prognosis. In the late 1990s and early 2000s, retrospective studies reported improved neurologic outcomes after CA with therapeutic hypothermia (TH), possibly due to reduced cerebral oxygen consumption.

OBJECTIVES
To determine if TH improves neurologic outcomes in nonresponsive patients after CA.

METHODS
Randomized trial with blinded assessment at 9 European centers from 1996 to 2001.

Patients
275 patients with return of spontaneous circulation (ROSC) after witnessed out-of-hospital CA. Inclusion criteria included a presumed cardiac etiology, age 18 to 75 years, shockable initial rhythm, 5 to 15 minutes from arrest to initiation of professional resuscitation, and <60 minutes from collapse to ROSC. Exclusion criteria included antecedent terminal illness, responsiveness to commands after ROSC, and persistent hypotension or hypoxia after ROSC.

Intervention
Hypothermia (with target temperature 32° to 34°C using external cooling mattress device and ice packs, maintained for 24 hours and followed by passive rewarming) versus control (maintenance of normothermia).

Outcomes
The primary outcome was favorable neurologic status (defined as category 1, "good recovery," or category 2, "moderate disability," on the 5-category Pittsburgh cerebral performance scale) at 6 months. Secondary endpoints included 6-month mortality and rate of complications.

KEY RESULTS

- More patients in the hypothermia group achieved favorable neurologic status (55% vs. 39%, RR 1.40, 95% CI 1.08–1.81, $p = 0.009$).
- 6-month mortality was lower among patients receiving TH (41% vs. 55%, RR 0.74, 95% CI 0.58–0.95, $p = 0.02$).
- There were no statistically significant differences between groups in overall complications, bleeding, or sepsis.

STUDY CONCLUSIONS

Among patients with ROSC and unresponsiveness after witnessed out-of-hospital CA with initial shockable rhythm; TH to 32° to 34°C improved neurologic outcomes and lowered mortality.

COMMENTARY

Together with a smaller, simultaneously published study that reported similar results, HACA produced the first randomized evidence evaluating TH in survivors of CA. It found striking effect sizes: the number needed to treat was only 6 to prevent unfavorable neurologic outcome, and only 7 to save a life. Results should be interpreted in view of two caveats. First, the protocol excluded nonshockable initial cardiac rhythms, limiting generalizability. Second, many patients in the control group developed temperatures >37°C, making it impossible to distinguish whether the primary benefit of cooling was achievement of lower temperature or avoidance of high temperature. A subsequent study[1] randomized nonresponsive patients after out-of-hospital CA (including shockable and nonshockable initial cardiac rhythms) to TH at 33°C or 36°C while avoiding temperatures >37°C in both groups. It found no difference in mortality or neurologic outcomes between groups, suggesting that avoidance of high temperatures may be the primary benefit. Accordingly, the 2015 American Heart Association post arrest care guidelines recommend TH to a target temperature range of 32° to 36°C regardless of initial cardiac rhythm.

Question

Should patients with ROSC and unresponsiveness after CA undergo temperature management?

Answer

Yes, cooling to target temperature of 32° to 36°C, and avoidance of temperatures >37°C, improves neurologic outcomes and lowers mortality.

References

1. Nielsen N, Wetterslev J, Cronberg T, et al; TTM Trial Investigators. Targeted temperature management at 33°C versus 36°C after cardiac arrest. *N Engl J Med.* 2013;369(23):2197–2206.

CHAPTER 23

CORTICOSTEROIDS IN SEPTIC SHOCK: THE CORTICUS TRIAL

Jessica Lee-Pancoast

Hydrocortisone Therapy for Patients With Septic Shock

Sprung CL, Annane D, Keh D, et al. *N Engl J Med*. 2008;358(2):111–124

BACKGROUND

Prior to this study, low-dose adjuvant corticosteroids in septic shock became standard therapy after a French trial demonstrated a substantial survival benefit among those with relative adrenal insufficiency.[1]

OBJECTIVES

To assess whether low-dose hydrocortisone improves mortality in patients with septic shock and variable degrees of baseline adrenal responsiveness.

METHODS

Randomized, double-blind, placebo-controlled trial at 52 sites in 9 countries in Europe and the Middle East between 2002 and 2005.

Patients

499 patients. Inclusion criteria included age ≥18 years, infection with systemic response and recent (within previous 72 hours) onset of shock (need for vasopressors or hypotension despite adequate fluid resuscitation) and sepsis-related organ dysfunction or hypoperfusion. Exclusion criteria included underlying poor prognosis, immunosuppression, or recent corticosteroid use. Patients were stratified into 2 groups by response to corticotropin stimulation, with "responders" defined as those whose serum cortisol rose by >9 µg/dL.

Interventions

Hydrocortisone (50 mg intravenously every 6 hours for 5 days, followed by a 6-day taper) versus placebo.

Outcomes

The primary outcome was 28-day mortality among those with relative adrenal insufficiency (corticotropin nonresponders). Secondary outcomes included 28-day mortality among corticotropin responders and overall, reversal of shock, adverse events, and ICU, hospital, and 1-year mortality.

KEY RESULTS

- Among corticotropin nonresponders, there was no difference in 28-day mortality between hydrocortisone and placebo groups (39.2% vs. 36.1%, $p = 0.69$).
- There was no difference in mortality between treatment groups in responders ($p = 1.00$) or among all patients ($p = 0.51$).
- The proportion with shock reversal was similar in both groups in all patients; median time to reversal was shorter in the hydrocortisone group (3.3 days vs. 5.8 days, $p < 0.001$).
- Superinfection, including new sepsis or septic shock, was more common in the hydrocortisone group (OR 1.37; 95% CI 1.05–1.79).

STUDY CONCLUSIONS

Treatment with hydrocortisone did not reduce mortality regardless of corticotropin response, but did decrease the duration of shock. Therapy was associated with more superinfection and new episodes of sepsis.

COMMENTARY

CORTICUS showed corticosteroids should not be used routinely and cast doubt on the value of the corticotropin stimulation test in septic shock. Some argued that as a result of the French trial, the contemporary clinical practice of treating the most severely ill with corticosteroids led to enrollment of a relatively healthy study population, pointing to the trial's lower overall mortality and early termination from slow enrollment as evidence of sampling selection bias. The authors argued that the lower placebo group mortality was due instead to the study's different inclusion criteria. The combined impact of CORTICUS and the French trial (which may have identified a subset of early-onset, vasopressor-refractory patients who could benefit) is reflected in the 2012 Surviving Sepsis Campaign guidelines, which now recommend against routine corticosteroids, except when vasopressors are ineffective, and against the use of corticotropin testing in this setting.

Question

Should patients with septic shock be routinely treated with hydrocortisone?

Answer

No, hydrocortisone does not improve mortality, though it may reduce time to reversal of shock and be beneficial for those with vasopressor-refractory disease.

References

1. Annane D, Sébille V, Charpentier C, et al. Effect of treatment with low doses of hydrocortisone and fludrocortisone on mortality in patients with septic shock. *JAMA.* 2002;288(7):862–871.

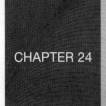

CHAPTER 24

LOW TIDAL VOLUME VENTILATION FOR ACUTE RESPIRATORY DISTRESS SYNDROME: THE ARMA TRIAL

Vivek T. Kulkarni

Ventilation With Lower Tidal Volumes as Compared With Traditional Tidal Volumes For Acute Lung Injury and the Acute Respiratory Distress Syndrome

The Acute Respiratory Distress Syndrome Network. *N Engl J Med*. 2000;342(18): 1301–1308

BACKGROUND

Prior to this study, acute respiratory distress syndrome (ARDS) carried a mortality rate of about 50%. Even significant advances in understanding its underlying mechanisms had not translated to effective treatment strategies. Animal models suggested a potential benefit of low tidal volume ventilation.

OBJECTIVES

To determine whether low tidal volume ventilation improves outcomes in patients with ARDS.

METHODS

Randomized controlled trial in 10 US centers between 1996 and 1999.

Patients

861 patients. Inclusion criteria included ARDS, defined by acute decrease in $PaO_2{:}FiO_2$ ratio to ≤ 300, bilateral pulmonary infiltrates, and lack of clinical evidence for left heart failure. Exclusion criteria included increased intracranial pressure, severe chronic respiratory disease, age <18 years, or presence of another condition with estimated 6-month mortality rate >50%.

Interventions

Low-volume ventilation (initial tidal volume of 6 cc/kg ideal body weight) versus traditional ventilation (initial tidal volume of 12 cc/kg ideal body weight). All patients received volume-assist-control ventilation. If plateau pressures were above goal (30 cm H_2O for low volume or 50 cm H_2O for traditional), tidal volume was decreased to a minimum of 4 cc/kg to achieve goal plateau pressures. Plateau pressure limits were liberalized if arterial pH fell below 7.15. FiO_2 and PEEP were adjusted to maintain PaO_2 55 to 80 mm Hg.

Outcomes

The first primary outcome was death in hospital or while still needing mechanical ventilation, up to 180 days. The second primary outcome was the number of ventilator-free days from days 1 to 28. Secondary outcomes included the number of days without nonpulmonary organ failure from days 1 to 28.

KEY RESULTS

- 180-day mortality was lower in the low-volume ventilation group (31.0% vs. 39.8%, $p = 0.007$).
- The low-volume ventilation group had more ventilator-free days (12 days vs. 10 days, $p = 0.007$).
- The low-volume ventilation group had a higher number of days without nonpulmonary organ failure (15 days vs. 12 days, $p = 0.006$).
- The incidence of barotrauma was similar between the 2 groups.

STUDY CONCLUSIONS

For patients with ARDS, low tidal volume ventilation lowers mortality and increases ventilator-free days and days without nonpulmonary organ failure.

COMMENTARY

Given the absolute mortality benefit of 8.8%, ARMA was terminated early. The study's protocol of low tidal volume ventilation conclusively demonstrated, for the first time, that a change in ventilator settings can dramatically improve outcomes in ARDS. Critics argued that the ventilation protocol between groups differed in more than just tidal volume; in particular, patients in the low-volume group were limited to lower plateau pressures and received higher PEEP. Some pointed out that the traditional group received more ventilation than was standard of care at the time, thereby increasing control group mortality. This study led to significant improvements in the treatment of a common and highly morbid condition. As a result, low tidal volume ventilation has become standard of care for patients with ARDS.

Question

Should patients with ARDS receive low tidal volume ventilation?

Answer

Yes, for patients with ARDS, low tidal volume ventilation lowers mortality, increases ventilator-free days, and increases days without nonpulmonary organ failure.

CHAPTER 25

TIMING OF ANTIBIOTICS IN SEPTIC SHOCK

Jessica Lee-Pancoast

Duration of Hypotension Before Initiation of Effective Antimicrobial Therapy Is the Critical Determinant of Survival in Human Septic Shock

Kumar A, Roberts D, Wood KE, et al. *Crit Care Med*. 2006;34(6):1589–1596

BACKGROUND

By the time of this study, early empiric (i.e., before microbiologic etiology had been established) antibiotic administration was standard practice for septic patients. Although a few studies had examined the effect of antibiotic timing from presentation or admission on outcomes, none had investigated the effect of antibiotic administration delays from the onset of key physiologic events, such as hypotension.

OBJECTIVES

To determine the relationship between timing of appropriate antimicrobial therapy in relation to hypotension onset and mortality in patients with septic shock.

METHODS

Retrospective cohort study of patients with diagnosis of septic shock from 1989 to 2004, drawing from academic and community intensive care units and hospitals in North America.

Patients

2,731 patients. Inclusion criteria were age ≥18 years and septic shock without other obvious cause of shock. Patients were included from the time they developed recurrent or persistent hypotension, defined as hypotension that persisted or only transiently improved after more than 2 Li of intravenous fluid resuscitation. 22% of cases involved suspected infection without identified pathogen or other confirmatory clinical evidence.

Interventions

Univariable and multivariable analyses with the primary predictor variable being time from first occurrence of persistent or recurrent hypotension to initiation of effective antimicrobial therapy (based either on sensitivities of isolated organisms or, if no organism was identified, on locally adapted guidelines for the clinical syndrome). Other independent variables included initial effectiveness of antibiotic therapy, type and degree of early fluid resuscitation, severity of illness, and type and timing of initial vasopressors.

Outcomes

The primary outcome was survival to hospital discharge.

KEY RESULTS

- Survival was 79.9% for patients who received appropriate antibiotics within the first hour of documented hypotension; over the first 6 hours, every hour of delay resulted in a mean 7.6% decrease in survival (range 3.6% to 9.9%).
- The relationship between survival and timing of effective antibiotic administration was present in all major subgroups (including by source of infection, culture positivity, and pathogen type).
- In multivariable analysis, timing of effective therapy was the strongest predictor of survival.

STUDY CONCLUSIONS

Delays in administration of effective antibiotics are associated with progressive increases in mortality.

COMMENTARY

This study had a major impact on the incorporation of antibiotic timing in key hospital quality metrics. Its large effect size has never been replicated, and some have questioned whether the critical window is truly 1 hour or a longer period of time. However, the relationship between antibiotics timing and survival has been confirmed in almost all subsequent studies. Furthermore, this study's robust dose–response curve supports causality, while its large and varied population implies generalizability. The 2012 Surviving Sepsis Campaign guidelines prominently cite this study to support a strong recommendation to administer effective intravenous antimicrobials within the first hour of recognition of severe sepsis and septic shock.

Question

Should patients with septic shock receive rapid and effective antibiotics?

Answer

Yes, delays in initiation of effective antimicrobial therapy are associated with increased mortality.

CHAPTER 26

PAIRED WEANING PROTOCOL FOR MECHANICAL VENTILATION AND SEDATION: THE ABC TRIAL

Vivek T. Kulkarni

Efficacy and Safety of a Paired Sedation and Ventilator Weaning Protocol for Mechanically Ventilated Patients in Intensive Care (Awakening and Breathing Controlled Trial): A Randomised Controlled Trial

Girard TD, Kress JP, Fuchs BD, et al. *Lancet.* 2008;371(9607):126–134

BACKGROUND

Mechanical ventilation frequently requires sedation, but sedative medications pose a challenge to ventilator weaning. Spontaneous awakening trials (SATs) that rely upon periodic interruption of sedative medications were a successful method to wean sedation. Researchers had also shown benefits from spontaneous breathing trials (SBTs) whereby ventilated patients intermittently received minimal ventilatory support to assess their readiness for weaning and extubation. Studies assessing these potentially synergistic strategies together were lacking.

OBJECTIVES

To assess the safety and efficacy of a protocol of paired SATs and SBTs versus SBTs alone.

METHODS

Randomized controlled trial at 4 US centers from 2003 to 2006.

Patients

336 patients. Inclusion criteria included need for mechanical ventilation for ≥12 hours and age ≥18 years. Exclusion criteria included admission for cardiac arrest, imminent death, profound neurologic deficits, and continuous mechanical ventilation for ≥2 weeks.

Interventions

Paired weaning versus control. In the paired weaning group, patients who met daily SAT safety requirements (including absence of seizures and alcohol withdrawal, nonescalating sedative dose, and no neuromuscular blockade) underwent SAT (interruption of all sedatives for up to 4 hours).

Those who failed were restarted on sedatives at half the previous dose, titrated to patient comfort. Those who passed underwent SBT barring contraindication (including inadequate oxygenation, lack of spontaneous inspiratory effort, or significant vasopressor support); physicians of patients who passed SBT were notified, while patients who failed immediately resumed prior ventilatory support; the decision of when or whether to extubate was left to the clinical team. The control group underwent only the SBT portion of the protocol. All patients received sedation to a clinically appropriate level of arousal.

Outcomes

The primary outcome was the number of ventilator-free days from day 1 to 28 (patients who died were considered to have 0 ventilator-free days). Secondary outcomes included time to ICU discharge, 28-day mortality, and 1-year mortality.

KEY RESULTS

- The paired weaning group had more ventilator-free days (14.7 days vs. 11.6 days, $p = 0.02$).
- Time to ICU discharge was shorter in the paired weaning group (9.1 days vs. 12.9 days, $p = 0.01$).
- While there were no statistically significant differences in 28-day mortality (28% in paired weaning group vs. 35% in control, $p = 0.21$), 1-year mortality was lower in the paired weaning group (44% vs. 58%, $p = 0.01$).

STUDY CONCLUSIONS

Compared with patients who received an SBT-only protocol, patients who received a protocol of daily SATs and SBTs experienced more ventilator-free days, earlier ICU discharge, and lower 1-year mortality.

COMMENTARY

ABC demonstrated impressive outcomes by pairing weaning protocols. It was large and well performed, and the simplicity of its protocol allowed for easy extension into most ICUs. The study was criticized because patients did not receive protocolized sedative dosing, and subsequent work showed that daily sedation interruption did not affect outcomes in the presence of a sedation protocol. Although the ideal strategy to manage sedation remains unknown, ABC and other trials support the notion that minimization of sedatives and daily assessment of extubation readiness improve outcomes. Accordingly, the 2013 Society of Critical Care Medicine pain, agitation, and delirium guidelines recommend either daily sedation interruption or protocolized sedation routinely in mechanically ventilated adults.

Question

Should mechanically ventilated patients undergo early and daily awakening and extubation readiness assessments?

Answer

Yes, in the absence of a sedation protocol, the addition of SATs to SBTs results in more ventilator-free days, earlier ICU discharge, and lower mortality.

CHAPTER 27

BLOOD TRANSFUSION FOR ICU PATIENTS: THE TRICC TRIAL

Viswatej Avutu

A Multicenter, Randomized, Controlled Clinical Trial of Transfusion Requirements in Critical Care.

Hébert PC, Wells G, Blajchman MA, et al. *N Engl J Med*. 1999;340(6):409–417

BACKGROUND

At the time of this study, most guidelines promoted a hemoglobin (Hgb) threshold of 10.0 g/dL as a general indication for transfusion in critically ill patients, based on small and/or narrowly focused (e.g., sickle cell patients) studies. Although anemia may not be well tolerated by these patients, they were also felt to be particularly susceptible to transfusion-related complications. Amid these trade-offs, the optimal transfusion practice for critically ill patients had not been established.

OBJECTIVES

To determine whether a restrictive red blood cell transfusion strategy is equivalent to a more liberal strategy in critically ill patients.

METHODS

Randomized, controlled equivalency trial in 25 Canadian intensive care units (ICUs) between 1994 and 1997. Randomization was stratified by disease severity as assessed by the Acute Physiology and Chronic Health Evaluation (APACHE) II score.

Patients

838 patients. Inclusion criteria included age ≥16 years, expected ICU stay >24 hours, Hgb ≤9 g/dL within 72 hours of ICU admission, and euvolemia after initial resuscitation. Exclusion criteria included ICU admission after routine cardiac surgical procedure, inability to receive blood products, active blood loss at the time of enrollment, chronic anemia, or imminent death.

Interventions

Restrictive (Hgb threshold of 7.0 g/dL; maintenance between 7.0 and 9.0 g/dL) versus liberal (Hgb threshold of 10.0 g/dL; maintenance between 10.0 and 12.0 g/dL) transfusion strategy.

Outcomes

The primary outcome was all-cause mortality at 30 days. Secondary outcomes included all-cause mortality at 60 days, and mortality rates during ICU and hospital stay. Lengths of stay and measures of organ failure and dysfunction were also assessed.

KEY RESULTS

- 30-day all-cause mortality was equivalent for the restrictive and liberal strategies overall (18.7% vs. 23.3%, $p = 0.11$), but was lower for the restrictive strategy among 2 subgroups: patients with APACHE II scores ≤ 20 (8.7% vs. 16.1%, $p = 0.03$) and patients <55 years old (5.7% vs. 13.0%, $p = 0.02$).
- There were no differences in 30-day all-cause mortality among subgroups by primary or secondary diagnosis (cardiac disease, severe infections and septic shock, or trauma).
- In-hospital mortality was lower in the restrictive strategy group, while cardiac complications during ICU stay were more frequent in the liberal strategy group.

STUDY CONCLUSIONS

A restrictive strategy is at least as effective as, and possibly superior to, a liberal strategy for red blood cell transfusion in most critically ill patients.

COMMENTARY

TRICC was important for providing evidence about the approach to red blood cell transfusion among critically ill patients. Caveats include a small proportion of patients with significant cardiac disease, which may limit application of study results to patients with acute myocardial infarction and unstable angina. Based on the TRICC results, the 2009 Society of Critical Care Medicine guidelines recommend a restrictive strategy for patients in the ICU.

Question

After initial resuscitation to euvolemia in critically ill patients, is a Hgb of 10.0 g/dL the ideal threshold for red blood cell transfusions?

Answer

No, in general a restrictive transfusion strategy (goal Hgb 7.0 to 9.0 g/dL) is at least as effective, and may be more effective in younger and less ill patients. However, clinicians should also consider patient-specific factors, particularly the presence of significant cardiac disease.

CHAPTER 28

CHOICE OF FIRST VASOPRESSOR IN SHOCK: THE SOAP II TRIAL

Vivek T. Kulkarni

Comparison of Dopamine and Norepinephrine in the Treatment of Shock

De Backer D, Biston P, Devriendt J, et al. *N Engl J Med*. 2010;362(9):779–789

BACKGROUND

Traditionally, dopamine and norepinephrine were both commonly used as initial vaso-pressors in patients with shock. Observational studies in the early 2000s began to suggest that dopamine may carry a higher risk of death, but randomized trials were too small to effectively guide therapy. At the time of this study, guidelines recommended either agent as first-line therapies.

OBJECTIVES

To determine whether the choice of norepinephrine or dopamine as a first vasopressor affects mortality in patients with shock.

METHODS

Randomized, double-blind, controlled trial in 8 European centers from 2003 to 2007.

Patients

1,679 patients. Inclusion criteria included shock (hypotension with tissue hypoperfusion) of any etiology requiring a vasopressor and age ≥ 18 years. Exclusion criteria included preceding vasopressor therapy for >4 hours, rapid atrial fibrillation (AF), and ventricular tachycardia (VT).

Interventions

Norepinephrine (0 to 0.19 µg/kg/min) versus dopamine (0 to 20 µg/kg/min) as a first vasopressor.

Outcomes

The primary outcome was 28-day mortality. Secondary outcomes included the rate of significant tachyarrhythmias. Outcomes were also assessed based on type of shock, which was a prespecified subgroup.

KEY RESULTS

- There was no statistically significant difference in 28-day mortality (52.5% in dopamine group vs. 48.5% in norepinephrine group, OR 1.17, 95% CI 0.97–1.42, $p = 0.10$).
- Among the 280 patients with cardiogenic shock, 28-day mortality was higher with dopamine ($p = 0.03$).
- Tachyarrhythmias occurred more frequently with dopamine (24.1% vs. 12.4%, $p < 0.001$), including AF (20.5% vs. 11.0%) and VT (2.4% vs. 1.0%).

STUDY CONCLUSIONS

Although the choice of norepinephrine or dopamine as first vasopressor had no significant impact on overall mortality, patients with cardiogenic shock had higher mortality with dopamine. Patients receiving dopamine also suffered more tachyarrhythmias.

COMMENTARY

SOAP II was the first large, double-blinded, and randomized trial to compare these commonly used first-line vasopressors. Additionally, because the inclusion criteria were broad, the results are readily generalizable. Despite the absence of a significant difference in overall mortality, patients receiving dopamine had an increased risk of tachyarrhythmias, which may explain the mortality difference in the prespecified cardiogenic shock subgroup (a group that may be particularly susceptible to the effects of tachyarrhythmia). A caveat is that the use of definitive therapies for shock (e.g., appropriate antibiotics in sepsis) was neither prospectively studied nor reported. The SOAP II findings have informed the 2012 Surviving Sepsis guidelines, which advocate for norepinephrine as the first vasopressor in septic shock, and the 2013 ACCF/AHA guidelines on ST-elevation myocardial infarction, which now caution that dopamine may be hazardous in cardiogenic shock.

Question

Is it reasonable to choose norepinephrine over dopamine as a first vasopressor in shock?

Answer

Yes, compared with dopamine, norepinephrine is associated with a lower risk of tachyarrhythmia in all types of shock. In patients with cardiogenic shock, it is associated with lower mortality.

CHAPTER 29

REVASCULARIZATION FOR CARDIOGENIC SHOCK AFTER MYOCARDIAL INFARCTION: THE SHOCK TRIAL

Vivek T. Kulkarni

Early Revascularization in Acute Myocardial Infarction Complicated by Cardiogenic Shock. SHOCK Investigators.

Hochman JS, Sleeper LA, Webb JG, et al. *N Engl J Med*. 1999;341(9):625–634

BACKGROUND

Prior to this trial, nonrandomized studies had suggested that early coronary revascularization after acute myocardial infarction (AMI) could reduce the significant morbidity from subsequent cardiogenic shock. The only randomized trial was inconclusive because of small size and early termination from low enrollment.

OBJECTIVES

To evaluate whether emergent revascularization for post-AMI cardiogenic shock improves mortality.

METHODS

Randomized trial across 30 centers in North America, South America, Australia, and Europe between 1993 and 1998.

Patients

302 patients. Inclusion criteria included AMI with ST elevation (including new left bundle branch block or posterior infarction with anterior ST depression) or Q waves, with clinical and hemodynamic evidence for cardiogenic shock. Exclusion criteria included severe systemic illness, severe valvular disease, mechanical etiology of shock, or unsuitability for revascularization.

Interventions

Emergent revascularization (within 6 hours, via either coronary artery bypass graft surgery or percutaneous coronary intervention, with increasing use of stents over the course of the trial) versus medical stabilization (recommended to receive immediate thrombolytic therapy, optimal medical therapy, and optional revascularization after 54 hours). All patients were recommended to receive intra-aortic balloon counterpulsation.

Outcomes

The primary outcome was 30-day mortality. Secondary outcomes included 6-month mortality.

KEY RESULTS

- There was no statistically significant difference in 30-day mortality between the two groups (46.7% in the emergent revascularization group vs. 56.0% in the medical stabilization group, RR 0.83, 95% CI 0.67–1.04, p = 0.11).
- 6-month mortality was lower among the emergent revascularization group (50.3% vs. 63.1%, RR 0.80, 95% CI 0.65–0.98, p = 0.027).
- Patients <75 years old (a prespecified subgroup) had lower 30-day mortality with emergent revascularization (RR 0.73, 95% CI 0.56–0.95, p = 0.02), while older patients had no statistically significant difference in mortality (RR 1.41, 95% 0.95–2.11, p = 0.16).

STUDY CONCLUSIONS

For patients with post-AMI cardiogenic shock, emergent coronary revascularization did not significantly lower 30-day mortality, but did lower 6-month mortality.

COMMENTARY

SHOCK was the first large randomized trial to assess the impact of emergent revascularization on post-AMI cardiogenic shock. It was criticized for failing to achieve a statistically significant primary outcome, though the difference in the secondary outcome, continued separation of survival curves, and confirmation from 1- and 6-year follow-up studies collectively support the significant, long-lived benefits of emergent revascularization. Based in large part on SHOCK, the 2013 ACCF/AHA guidelines on ST-elevation myocardial infarction recommend emergent revascularization for post-AMI cardiogenic shock in patients under 75, and consider it "reasonable" in patients over 75.

Question

Should patients with post-AMI cardiogenic shock undergo emergent coronary revascularization?

Answer

Yes, emergent coronary revascularization lowers long-term mortality in patients with post-AMI cardiogenic shock.

CHAPTER 30

EARLY GOAL-DIRECTED THERAPY IN SEPSIS

Jessica Lee-Pancoast

Early Goal-Directed Therapy in the Treatment of Severe Sepsis and Septic Shock
Rivers E, Nguyen B, Havstad S, et al. *N Engl J Med*. 2001;345(19):1368–1377

BACKGROUND
Prior to this study, numerous severe sepsis and septic shock intervention trials in the intensive care unit were at best only marginally successful, and mortality from these common conditions remained high. It was unknown whether earlier interventions to optimize physiologic variables could improve survival.

OBJECTIVES
To determine if early goal-directed therapy (EGDT) delivered in the emergency room before admission reduces mortality among patients with severe sepsis or septic shock.

METHODS
Randomized controlled trial in a single American emergency room from 1997 to 2000.

Patients
263 patients. Inclusion criteria included ≥ 2 systemic inflammatory response syndrome criteria and either SBP ≤ 90 mm Hg after initial fluid challenge or blood lactate ≥ 4 mmol/L. Exclusion criteria included age <18 years, acute stroke or coronary syndrome, pulmonary edema, cancer on chemotherapy, or immunosuppression.

Interventions
EGDT versus standard therapy. EGDT consisted of the following sequential goals in the first 6 hours of treatment: fluid boluses every 30 minutes to maintain CVP 8 to 12 mm Hg; vasodilators or vasopressors to maintain MAP 65 to 90 mm Hg; and blood transfusion (until hematocrit $\geq 30\%$) and dobutamine to maintain continuously monitored $ScvO_2$ $\geq 70\%$. Sedation and mechanical ventilation were used as necessary. Standard therapy consisted of maintaining, at the clinicians' discretion, CVP 8 to 12 mm Hg, urine output ≥ 0.5 mL/kg/hr, and MAP ≥ 65 mm Hg.

Outcomes
The primary outcome was in-hospital mortality. Secondary outcomes included 28- and 60-day mortality and treatments administered.

KEY RESULTS

- EGDT led to lower in-hospital mortality (30.5% vs. 46.5%, RR 0.58; 95% CI 0.38–0.87, $p = 0.009$) and mortality at 28 days (RR 0.58; 95% CI 0.39–0.87) and 60 days (RR 0.67; 95% CI 0.46–0.96).
- In the first 6 hours, EGDT patients received more fluid (5.0 L vs. 3.5 L, $p < 0.001$), blood transfusions ($p < 0.001$), and dobutamine ($p < 0.001$) than standard therapy patients.
- By 72 hours, standard treatment patients had received similar amounts of fluid ($p = 0.73$) but were more likely to be on vasopressors ($p = 0.02$) and mechanical ventilation ($p = 0.02$).

STUDY CONCLUSIONS

EGDT improves outcomes among patients with severe sepsis and septic shock.

COMMENTARY

The mortality reduction reported in this study was seminal to the creation of the Surviving Sepsis Campaign, which recommended EGDT for initial management. Efforts to incorporate EGDT as the standard of care, however, have been limited by several concerns: the trial's very high mortality and potentially nongeneralizable population, as well as the protocol's bundled nature and the resultant difficulty identifying which specific interventions were beneficial. Some components of EGDT – use of CVP as the sole marker of volume responsiveness, aggressive use of blood transfusion and inotropes, reliance on expensive and invasive continuous $ScvO_2$ monitoring – were not supported in subsequent investigations. Furthermore, a meta-analysis[1] that included 3 recent, large, multicentered, harmonized clinical trials (ProCESS, ARISE/ANZICS, and ProMISe) showed no benefit for EGDT over contemporary, nonprotocolized usual care, and the role of a formal algorithm is now questionable. One possible interpretation of these discordant results is that "usual care" has evolved significantly with respect to fluid resuscitation practices in large part due to the original EGDT trial, which clearly established the value of early and aggressive fluids with close hemodynamic monitoring.

Question

Does EGDT reduce mortality among patients with severe sepsis or septic shock?

Answer

No, several aspects of EGDT are of unclear benefit, but early and aggressive fluid resuscitation with frequent monitoring remain key aspects of the standard of care.

References

1. Angus DC, Barnato AE, Bell D, et al. A systematic review and meta-analysis of early goal-directed therapy for septic shock: The ARISE, ProCESS and ProMISe Investigators. *Intensive Care Med.* 2015;41(9):1549–1560.

CHAPTER 31

PRONE POSITIONING IN SEVERE ARDS: THE PROSEVA TRIAL

Jessica Lee-Pancoast

Prone Positioning in Severe Acute Respiratory Distress Syndrome

Guérin C, Reignier J, Richard JC, et al. *N Engl J Med*. 2013;368(23):2159–2168

BACKGROUND

Prior to this study, prone positioning had been shown to improve physiologic measures, such as oxygenation, for patients with acute respiratory distress syndrome (ARDS). Though meta-analyses suggested a survival benefit, no previous randomized trial had demonstrated such an outcome. Moreover, the optimal timing and duration of proning was unknown.

OBJECTIVES

To evaluate the effect of early and prolonged application of prone positioning in patients with severe ARDS.

METHODS

Randomized controlled trial of 466 patients in 27 European intensive care units (ICUs) from 2008 to 2011.

Patients

466 adult patients. Inclusion criteria included severe ARDS with <36 hours of mechanical ventilation. In addition to the general Consensus Criteria definition for ARDS, severe disease was defined as a PaO_2:FiO_2 ratio <150 mm Hg, with FiO_2 ≥0.6, PEEP ≥5 cm H_2O, and tidal volume of approximately 6 mL/kg predicted body weight. Exclusion criteria included elevated intracranial pressure, mean arterial pressure <65 mm Hg, acute deep vein thrombosis, and other diseases resulting in a life expectancy <1 year. At randomization, the proning group had a higher rate of neuromuscular blockade, while the supine group had greater use of vasopressor agents and higher organ dysfunction scores. The groups were otherwise well balanced.

Interventions

Prone (proned within 1 hour after randomization and maintained for ≥16 consecutive hours, with proning stopped for significantly improved or worsened oxygenation, or for severe complications such as cardiac arrest or unscheduled extubation) for 28 days versus supine (maintained in semirecumbent position) position strategy. All patients received a standardized lung protective strategy with low tidal volumes and frequent use of neuromuscular blockade.

Outcomes

The primary outcome was 28-day mortality. Secondary outcomes included 90-day mortality, rates of successful extubation, length of ICU stay, and complications.

KEY RESULTS

- 28-day mortality was lower in the prone group (16.0% vs. 32.8%, HR 0.39, 95% CI 0.25–0.63, $p < 0.001$). This difference persisted after adjustment for baseline organ dysfunction score, neuromuscular blockade, and vasopressor use.
- The prone group had lower mortality at day 90 (23.6% vs. 41.0%, HR 0.44, 95% CI 0.29–0.67, $p < 0.001$).
- More prone patients were successfully extubated by day 90 (80.5% vs. 65.0%, HR 0.45, 95% CI 0.29–0.70, $p < 0.001$).
- There were no statistically significant differences between the two groups in duration of mechanical ventilation or length of ICU stay.
- There were more cardiac arrests among supine patients (31 vs. 16, $p = 0.02$), but otherwise no statistically significant differences in complications.

STUDY CONCLUSIONS

Patients with severe ARDS benefit from prone positioning when it is applied early and for relatively long sessions.

COMMENTARY

PROSEVA demonstrated a remarkable survival benefit for prone positioning. It differed from previous trials in that it targeted patients with more severe hypoxemia, and involved proning earlier and for longer periods. Caveats include the low rate of procedural complications (likely due to prior proning experience at study sites) and baseline patient imbalances, especially in the use of neuromuscular blockade. Since PROSEVA's publication, the use of prone positioning for severe ARDS has increased significantly.

Question

Should patients with severe ARDS be proned?

Answer

Yes, early and extended prone positioning in experienced centers has been shown to reduce mortality.

ENDOCRINOLOGY

CHAPTER 32

ACE INHIBITORS FOR DIABETIC NEPHROPATHY

Melissa G. Lechner

The Effect of Angiotensin-Converting-Enzyme Inhibition on Diabetic Nephropathy
Lewis EJ, Hunsicker LG, Bain RP, et al. *N Engl J Med*. 1993;329(20):1456–1462

BACKGROUND
Renal disease is recognized as a significant sequela of diabetes mellitus and hypertension. Prior studies had shown that treatment of hypertension slowed progression of kidney disease in patients with diabetic nephropathy. Additionally, data from animal models suggested that angiotensin-converting-enzyme (ACE) inhibitors could provide renal protection and reduce glomerular damage via mechanisms that were independent of their blood pressure effects.

OBJECTIVES
To determine whether the ACE inhibitor captopril is more effective in slowing the progression of diabetic nephropathy than other antihypertensive agents.

METHODS
Randomized, double-blind, controlled trial at 30 centers between 1987 and 1990.

Patients
409 patients with or without pre-existing hypertension. Inclusion criteria included age 18 to 49 years, insulin-dependent diabetes mellitus (IDDM) for ≥7 years with onset before age 30 and complicated by retinopathy and proteinuria (≥500 mg/day). Exclusion criteria included serum creatinine >2.5 mg/dL, hyperkalemia, severe heart failure, and pregnancy. At baseline, patients in the placebo group had higher urinary protein excretion than those in the captopril group ($p = 0.02$).

Interventions
Captopril (25 mg 3 times daily) versus placebo. Blood pressure was titrated to systolic blood pressure (SBP) <140 mm Hg and diastolic blood pressure (DBP) <90 mm Hg; if SBP >150 mm Hg at baseline, titrated to a decrease in SBP by 10 mm Hg or maximal SBP <160 mm Hg. All patients received conventional diabetes management as well as blood pressure treatment with other classes of medications, including diuretics, beta-adrenergic antagonists, clonidine, methyldopa, and hydralazine. Treatment with calcium channel blockers outside of the study intervention was not allowed.

Outcomes
The primary outcome was doubling of serum creatinine to ≥2 mg/dL. Secondary outcomes included urinary protein excretion, 24-hour creatinine clearance, and cumulative incidence of death, need for dialysis or renal transplant.

KEY RESULTS

- Fewer patients receiving captopril experienced doubling of serum creatinine (25 vs. 43, p = 0.007) with a risk reduction of 43% (95% CI 6%–65%) after adjusting for mean arterial blood pressure.
- After adjustment for mean arterial blood pressure, captopril was associated with a reduction in the cumulative incidence of death, need for dialysis, or renal transplant by 46% (95% CI 10%–68%).
- Risk reductions for both outcomes were more pronounced in subgroups with worse baseline renal function (serum creatinine ≥1.5 mg/dL).

STUDY CONCLUSIONS

Captopril protects against deterioration in renal function in patients with IDDM complicated by retinopathy and nephropathy and is more effective than blood pressure control alone.

COMMENTARY

This study established the renoprotective effects of ACE inhibitors in patients with diabetes mellitus and nephropathy. Caveats include a high proportion of white patients and those with poorly controlled disease (baseline hemoglobin A1c >11%), the use of urinary protein loss and creatinine clearance as surrogate markers of renal function, and imbalance between groups in baseline urinary protein excretion. Subsequent studies corroborated the renal and cardiovascular benefits of ACE inhibitors in other diabetic populations, collectively informing the 2016 ADA Standards of Medical Care recommendations to use ACE inhibitors as first-line antihypertensive agents in diabetic patients.

Question

Should patients with diabetic nephropathy be treated with ACE inhibitors?

Answer

Yes, ACE inhibitors have renoprotective effects independent of blood pressure control.

CHAPTER 33

BISPHOSPHONATES AND FRACTURE RISK: THE FIT TRIAL

Melissa G. Lechner

Effect of Alendronate on Risk of Fracture in Women With Low Bone Density but Without Vertebral Fractures

Cummings SR, Black DM, Thompson DE, et al. *JAMA*. 1998;280(24):2077–2082

BACKGROUND

To evaluate the benefits of bisphosphonate therapy in postmenopausal women with low bone mineral density (BMD), earlier analyses from the FIT investigators had demonstrated that alendronate reduces fracture risk among women with prior vertebral fracture. However, the vast majority of postmenopausal women with low BMD have never suffered prior vertebral fractures. The effect of bisphosphonates on fracture risk among these women remained unknown.

OBJECTIVES

To test whether alendronate would decrease the risk of clinical fractures in women with low BMD but no prior vertebral fractures.

METHODS

Randomized, double-blind, placebo-controlled trial in 11 US clinical centers between 1992 and 1997.

Patients

4,432 female patients. Inclusion criteria included age 55 to 80 years, postmenopausal status for ≥ 2 years, BMD ≥ 1.6 standard deviations below the normal young adult mean (i.e., T-score −1.6 or lower), and no prior vertebral fracture. Exclusion criteria included significant renal or liver disease, thyroid disease, hyperparathyroidism, severe malabsorption, and recent calcitonin or estrogen therapy. At baseline, 37% of patients had baseline osteoporosis (T-score −2.5 or lower).

Interventions

Alendronate (5 mg/day, increased to 10 mg/day after the second annual visit based on contemporary trials suggesting this dose had greater effects on BMD) versus placebo. All women with low dietary calcium also received daily calcium (500 mg elemental) and vitamin D supplementation (250 IU). Patients were treated for 4 years.

Outcomes

The primary outcome was clinical fractures, defined as nontraumatic fractures diagnosed by physicians and confirmed on radiography. Other outcomes included new vertebral deformity (fracture detected on radiography) and BMD (detected on dual x-ray absorptiometry). Adverse events included gastrointestinal problems (e.g., esophagitis, ulcers).

KEY RESULTS

- There was no statistically significant difference in the overall incidence of clinical fractures (12.3% in the alendronate group vs. 14.1% in placebo group, relative hazard 0.86, 95% CI 0.73–1.01).
- Alendronate increased BMD at all anatomic sites measured ($p < 0.001$).
- Among women with baseline femoral neck osteoporosis (BMD >2.5 standard deviations below the normal young adult mean), alendronate was associated with lower incidence of clinical fractures (13.1% vs. 19.6%, relative hazard 0.64, 95% CI 0.50–0.82).
- Patients receiving alendronate had lower incidence of new vertebral deformities (2.1% vs. 3.8%, RR 0.56, 95% CI 0.39–0.80).
- There were no statistically significant differences between groups with respect to discontinuation of study medication or rates of death or gastrointestinal problems.

STUDY CONCLUSIONS

In postmenopausal women with low BMD and no prior vertebral fractures, alendronate increased BMD and reduced the risk of vertebral deformity. It also reduced the risk of clinical fractures among osteoporotic women but not those with higher BMD.

COMMENTARY

This analysis from the FIT trial answered a question of great relevance to the majority of postmenopausal women with low BMD. Of note, it did not assess the adequacy of vitamin D supplementation or include women on estrogen therapy, though 10% of participants in both groups received estrogen for some period. Along with subsequent work, the results of this study have informed the 2014 National Osteoporosis Foundation recommendation to initiate bisphosphonate therapy in patients with prior vertebral fracture, osteoporosis defined by low BMD (T-scores ≤–2.5), or osteopenia (T-score –1.0 to –2.5) and a ≥3% 10-year hip fracture risk or a ≥20% 10-year major osteoporosis-related fracture risk as determined by the US-adapted World Health Organization absolute fracture risk model (Fracture Risk Algorithm [FRAX®]).

Question

Should postmenopausal women with femoral neck BMD –2.6 standard deviations from the normal young adult mean receive bisphosphonates?

Answer

Yes, even among those without prior vertebral fracture, bisphosphonate treatment reduces clinical fractures and vertebral deformities in these patients.

CHAPTER 34

INSULIN THERAPY AND DIABETES COMPLICATIONS: THE DCCT TRIAL

Melissa G. Lechner

The Effect of Intensive Treatment of Diabetes on the Development and Progression of Long-Term Complications in Insulin-Dependent Diabetes Mellitus

The Diabetes Control and Complications Trial Research Group. *N Engl J Med*. 1993; 329(14):977–986

BACKGROUND

At the time of this study, the long-term risks of diabetes mellitus were well recognized. Epidemiologic and animal studies implicated hyperglycemia in disease pathogenesis, but causal relationships were unproven in humans and it was unclear whether glycemic management through intensive insulin therapy could prevent or slow clinical complications. Earlier work had demonstrated that intensive therapy could delay the progression of microvascular disease among patients with insulin-dependent diabetes mellitus (IDDM) with poor glycemic control and retinopathy. However, data were lacking about whether it would provide similar benefits among patients with absent or only mild pre-existing complications.

OBJECTIVES

To determine if intensive insulin therapy can prevent or delay the progression of complications in patients with IDDM.

METHODS

Randomized controlled trial at 29 centers in the United States and Canada between 1983 and 1989.

Patients

1,441 patients. Inclusion criteria included age 13 to 39 years, IDDM (defined by deficient c-peptide secretion). Two cohorts were defined: a primary prevention group with a 1- to 5-year history of IDDM and no evidence of retinopathy, and a secondary prevention group with a 1- to 15-year history of IDDM and mild retinopathy.

Interventions

Intensive insulin therapy (via pump or ≥3 daily injections) versus standard therapy (via 1–2 daily injections). Patients were followed for a mean of 6.5 years.

Outcomes

The primary outcome in the primary prevention cohort was incident retinopathy. In the secondary prevention cohort, the primary outcome was the rate of progression of early retinopathy or the development of proliferative or severe retinopathy. Secondary outcomes in both cohorts included the rate of hypoglycemia and the development of cardiovascular disease, diabetic nephropathy, or diabetic neuropathy.

KEY RESULTS

- The average hemoglobin A1c (HgbA1c) was approximately 7% versus 9% in the intensive and standard therapy groups, respectively.
- Compared to standard therapy, intensive insulin therapy led to a 76% risk reduction in incident retinopathy (95% CI 62%–85%) in the primary prevention group, and a 54% risk reduction in the progression of retinopathy (95% CI 39%–66%) and 47% reduction in the development of proliferative or severe retinopathy (95% CI 14%–67%) in the secondary prevention group.
- Patients receiving intensive therapy also had reduced incidence of microalbuminuria, albuminuria, and neuropathy.
- Intensive insulin therapy was associated with a 3-fold higher incidence of severe hypoglycemia (62 vs. 19 episodes per 100 patient-years, $p < 0.001$).

STUDY CONCLUSIONS

In patients with IDDM, intensive insulin therapy delays the onset and slows the progression of retinopathy, nephropathy, and neuropathy compared with standard therapy.

COMMENTARY

DCCT was important for several reasons. First, it solidified the relationship between hyperglycemia and disease sequelae, showing that the risk of retinopathy fell continuously with declining HgbA1c and the risk of hypoglycemia increased continuously without a clear risk/benefit threshold. Second, its size and design allowed investigators to compare HgbA1c and serum glucose levels, ultimately validating HgbA1c as a proxy for glycemic control. Caveats include lack of significant clinical outcomes, such as renal failure and survival. Nonetheless, along with subsequent studies, DCCT helped define treatment goals supported by the 2016 American Diabetes Association Standards of Care in Diabetes.

Question

Is it reasonable to treat patients with IDDM to a target HgbA1c of 7%?

Answer

Yes, this approach can prevent or slow the development of microvascular complications for many adults, although these benefits should be weighed against the risk for hypoglycemia.

CHAPTER 35

HORMONE REPLACEMENT THERAPY IN POSTMENOPAUSAL WOMEN: THE WOMEN'S HEALTH INITIATIVE (WHI) TRIAL

Erik H. Knelson

Risks and Benefits of Estrogen Plus Progestin in Healthy Postmenopausal Women: principal Results From the Women's Health Initiative Randomized Controlled Trial.

Rossouw JE, Anderson GL, Prentice RL, et al. *JAMA.* 2002;288(3):321–333

BACKGROUND

Hormone replacement therapy (HRT) has traditionally been used primarily for the treatment of vasomotor symptoms in postmenopausal women. Prior to 2002, retrospective cohort studies and small clinical trials demonstrated an association between prolonged HRT and reduced risk of hip fracture, coronary artery disease (CAD), and hyperlipidemia, suggesting that it could be used for primary prevention of chronic disease in asymptomatic postmenopausal women.

OBJECTIVES

To assess the health benefits and risks of the most commonly used hormone replacement regimen in postmenopausal women.

METHODS

Randomized, double-blind, placebo-controlled, trial at 40 centers across the United States between 1993 and 1998.

Patients

16,608 women. Inclusion criteria included age 50 to 79 years with an intact uterus and postmenopausal status (no vaginal bleeding >6 months if age 55 to 79 years or >12 months if age 50 to 54 years). Exclusion criteria included predicted survival <3 years, history of breast cancer at any age or another cancer within 10 years, anemia, and thrombocytopenia.

Interventions

Daily combined HRT (estrogen 0.625 mg and medroxyprogesterone 2.5 mg) versus placebo. Patients were followed for a mean of 5.2 years, and dropout rates exceeded 35% in both groups.

Outcomes

The primary outcomes were CAD (defined as nonfatal MI or death from CAD) and invasive breast cancer. Secondary outcomes included stroke, pulmonary embolism (PE), endometrial and colorectal cancer, hip fracture, all-cause mortality, and a global index (a composite of primary and secondary outcomes, with a value >1 signifying increased risk).

KEY RESULTS

- HRT increased the risk of both CAD (HR 1.29, 95% CI 1.02–1.63) and breast cancer (HR 1.26, 95% CI 1.00–1.59).
- HRT increased the risk of stroke (HR 1.41, 95% CI 1.07–1.85) and PE (HR 2.13, 95% CI 1.39–3.25).
- HRT decreased the risk of colorectal cancer (HR 0.63, 95% CI 0.43–0.92) and hip fracture (HR 0.66, 95% CI 0.45–0.98).
- There were no statistically significant differences in endometrial cancer (HR 0.83, 95% CI 0.47–1.47) and all-cause mortality (HR 0.98, 95% CI 0.82–1.18).
- The global index was higher in the HRT group (HR 1.15, 95% CI 1.03–1.28).

STUDY CONCLUSIONS

The risks of hormone replacement outweigh the benefits for primary prevention of chronic disease in healthy postmenopausal women.

COMMENTARY

WHI called into question the long-term use of HRT in postmenopausal women for cardiac protection and cancer prevention. It was stopped early because the breast cancer risk exceeded a preset boundary and the global index demonstrated increased harm versus benefit. Caveats include an older population (mean age of 63), which potentially mitigated beneficial effects of HRT on the prevention of early coronary plaque formation, and the use of a relatively high dose of HRT. During WHI enrollment, the HERS study[1] demonstrated worsening of previously diagnosed CAD soon after initiation of HRT. Based on these trials, the 2012 US Preventive Services Task Force guidelines recommend against the use of HRT to prevent chronic conditions for postmenopausal women over age 50 without surgical menopause, but make no recommendations about HRT for the exclusive treatment of vasomotor symptoms.

Question

Should healthy postmenopausal women receive HRT to prevent chronic disease?

Answer

No, the risks of increased CAD, invasive breast cancer, stroke, and PE outweigh the benefits of decreased hip fractures and colorectal cancers.

References

1. Hulley S, Grady D, Bush T, et al. Randomized trial of estrogen plus progestin for secondary prevention of coronary heart disease in postmenopausal women. Heart and Estrogen/progestin Replacement Study (HERS) Research Group. *JAMA.* 1998;280(7):605–613.

CHAPTER 36

LIFESTYLE INTERVENTION AND METFORMIN IN DIABETES: THE DPP STUDY

Melissa G. Lechner

Reduction in the Incidence of Type 2 Diabetes with Lifestyle Intervention or Metformin

Diabetes Prevention Program Research Group. *N Engl J Med*. 2002;346(6):393–403

BACKGROUND

In the years leading up to this study, obesity, sedentary lifestyle, and poor diet were recognized as reversible risk factors for developing type 2 diabetes mellitus (T2DM). Observational studies had shown that exercise and healthy diet could prevent onset of T2DM in high-risk groups but did not examine the role of medications in prevention. The generalizability of these results to ethnically and culturally diverse populations also remained unclear.

OBJECTIVES

To evaluate the effectiveness of lifestyle intervention or treatment with metformin in preventing or delaying the development of T2DM in predisposed patients.

METHODS

Randomized controlled trial at 27 US centers between 1996 and 1999.

Patients

3,234 patients. Inclusion criteria included age ≥25 years, BMI ≥24 kg/m², blood glucose 95 to 125 mg/dL (fasting) and 140 to 199 mg/dL (2 hours after a glucose tolerance test). Exclusion criteria included use of medications known to increase or decrease blood glucose. The study aimed to enroll high percentages of minority populations.

Interventions

Metformin (850 mg twice daily) with standard lifestyle intervention versus placebo with standard lifestyle intervention versus intensive lifestyle modification. The standard lifestyle intervention consisted of written information and 1 annual 30-minute counseling session about weight loss and physical activity. Patients in the intensive modification group received a 16-lesson curriculum on diet and exercise with the goals of ≥7% weight reduction and ≥150 minutes of aerobic exercise per week. Participants were followed for a mean of 2.8 years.

Outcomes

The primary outcome was incident T2DM (via screening with annual glucose tolerance test and semiannual fasting blood glucose), measured in cases per 100 person-years.

KEY RESULTS

- Compared to those receiving placebo and standard lifestyle intervention, the incidence of T2DM was lower for patients receiving intensive lifestyle modification (4.8 vs. 11.0, risk reduction 58%, 95% CI 48%–66%) and metformin (7.8 vs. 11.0, risk reduction 31%, 95% CI 17%–43%).
- Intensive lifestyle modification led to a 39% risk reduction in incident T2DM (95% CI 24%–51%) compared to metformin.
- At 6 months, compliance in the intensive intervention group was 74% for exercise and 50% for weight loss goals.

STUDY CONCLUSIONS

Intensive lifestyle changes and treatment with metformin both reduced the diabetes incidence in persons at high risk, with lifestyle intervention being more effective than metformin.

COMMENTARY

Although generalizability to younger patients and those without impaired glucose tolerance may be limited, this study established the importance of structured lifestyle interventions in delaying or preventing T2DM in high-risk individuals. Importantly, the intervention was effective across different ethnic subpopulations, including African American, Hispanic, American Indian, and Asian groups, even in the setting of moderate compliance with exercise and weight loss goals. The efficacy of metformin also represents a key advancement. Based on study findings – including estimates that 1 case of T2DM could be avoided for every 7 patients undergoing intensive lifestyle modification or every 14 given metformin – the 2015 American Diabetes Association recommendations for preventing or delaying T2DM suggest consideration of both options.

Question

Should overweight patients with impaired fasting glucose and glucose intolerance receive intensive lifestyle interventions or metformin in order to prevent T2DM?

Answer

Yes, these patients should be referred to structured weight loss and exercise programs. Metformin can also be considered, although it has lower efficacy than lifestyle interventions.

GASTROENTEROLOGY

4

CHAPTER 37

ANTIBIOTICS IN VARICEAL GI BLEEDING

Nadim Mahmud

Systemic Antibiotic Therapy Prevents Bacterial Infection in Cirrhotic Patients With Gastrointestinal Hemorrhage

Blaise M, Pateron D, Trinchet J, et al. *Hepatology*. 1994;20(1):34–38

BACKGROUND

Cirrhotic patients are vulnerable to infection during acute gastrointestinal (GI) bleeding, as enteric bacterial translocation may occur during resuscitation or endoscopy. Gut decontamination regimens with nonabsorbed oral antibiotics had been shown to reduce infections in cirrhotic patients with GI hemorrhage. However, this approach relied upon an often-impractical oral route and did not address the added risk of translocation precipitated by endoscopy. No studies had evaluated systemic intravenous antibiotics prior to endoscopy.

OBJECTIVES

To evaluate the efficacy of early systemic ofloxacin and a pre-endoscopic amoxicillin/clavulanic acid (ACA) bolus in preventing bacterial infections in cirrhotic patients with variceal bleeding.

METHODS

Randomized controlled trial in a French hospital from 1990 to 1992.

Patients

91 patients. Inclusion criteria included cirrhosis, age >18 years, admission to the intensive care unit (ICU) for upper GI hemorrhage. Exclusion criteria included allergies to fluoroquinolones or beta-lactam antibiotics, absence of varices, recent antibiotics, or objective evidence of an established infection (assessed through urine, sputum, and blood cultures, chest x-ray, and diagnostic paracentesis).

Interventions

Ofloxacin (400 mg/day for 10 days) and ACA (1 g bolus prior to endoscopy) versus control (no prophylactic antibiotics). All patients underwent endoscopy within 12 hours of admission, with patients routinely evaluated for infection in a manner analogous to the initial infectious workup.

Outcomes

The primary outcome was occurrence of infection through 14 days of hospitalization. Secondary outcomes included 14-day mortality, length of ICU stay, number of blood transfusions, and recurrent hemorrhage.

KEY RESULTS
- The rate of infections at 14 days was lower in patients receiving early systemic antibiotics (19.6% vs. 66.7%, $p < 0.001$).
- There was no statistically significant difference in 14-day mortality between the groups (23.9% vs. 35.6%).
- There were no statistically significant differences between groups in length of ICU stay, number of blood transfusions, or recurrent hemorrhage.

STUDY CONCLUSIONS
In cirrhotic patients with variceal bleeding, prophylactic systemic antibiotic therapy with ofloxacin and a pre-endoscopic ACA bolus reduces the rate of bacterial infection.

COMMENTARY

This was the first study to demonstrate a marked reduction in infections with systemic intravenous antibiotics in cirrhotic patients with variceal bleeding. Some major caveats inherent to the trial design were that the study was not placebo controlled, and the relative contributions of ofloxacin and ACA could not be determined. Nevertheless, this and subsequent studies established experimental evidence supporting prophylactic antibiotics, in particular fluoroquinolones, to prevent enteric bacterial translocation in this population. Importantly, although this study did not detect a mortality benefit, this was later demonstrated through meta-analysis.[1] These contributions are reflected in the 2007 American Association for the Study of Liver Diseases variceal guidelines, which recommend preventive oral norfloxacin, intravenous ciprofloxacin, or intravenous ceftriaxone in cirrhotic patients with variceal hemorrhage.

Question
Should cirrhotic patients with variceal bleeding receive early prophylactic antibiotics?

Answer
Yes, antibiotics started on presentation of variceal bleeding reduce infection and mortality.

References
1. Bernard B, Grangé JD, Khac EN, et al. Antibiotic prophylaxis for the prevention of bacterial infections in cirrhotic patients with gastrointestinal bleeding: a meta-analysis. *Hepatology.* 1999;29(6):1655–1661.

CHAPTER 38

TRANSFUSION IN UGIB

Nadim Mahmud

Transfusion Strategies for Acute Upper Gastrointestinal Bleeding
Villanueva C, Colomo A, Bosch A, et al. *N Engl J Med*. 2013;368(1):11–21

BACKGROUND

At the time of this study, there was great uncertainty surrounding appropriate hemoglobin (Hgb) transfusion thresholds in patients with acute upper gastrointestinal bleeding (UGIB). Although literature from the critical care setting found restrictive transfusion to be at least as effective as liberal transfusion, patients with GI bleeding were often excluded from these investigations. In fact, several small studies suggested possible harm from transfusions in patients with UGIB.

OBJECTIVES

To determine if restrictive red cell transfusion was safer and more effective than liberal transfusion in patients with acute UGIB.

METHODS

Randomized, controlled trial at a single Spanish hospital between 2003 and 2009.

Patients

921 patients with hematemesis, melena, or both. Inclusion criteria included age >18 years. Exclusion criteria included massive exsanguinating bleeding, lower GI bleeding, very low-risk GI bleeding (per the Rockall score and baseline Hgb), and recent trauma, surgery, or vascular events (e.g., acute coronary syndrome, transient ischemic attack, or stroke).

Interventions

Restrictive (Hgb threshold of 7 g/dL; maintenance between 7 and 9 g/dL) versus liberal (Hgb threshold of 9 g/dL; maintenance between 9 and 11 g/dL) transfusion strategy. All patients underwent upper endoscopy within 6 hours.

Outcomes

The primary outcome was the rate of all-cause mortality within the first 45 days. Secondary outcomes included the rate of in-hospital complications and the rate of further bleeding.

KEY RESULTS

- Patients treated with a restrictive transfusion strategy had a lower 45-day mortality rate (5% vs. 9%, $p = 0.02$).
- Rates of complications were significantly lower in the restrictive strategy group (40% vs. 48%, $p = 0.02$).
- Rates of further bleeding were significantly lower in the restrictive strategy group (10% vs. 16%, $p = 0.01$).

STUDY CONCLUSIONS

Among patients presenting with severe acute UGIB, a restrictive transfusion strategy (goal Hgb >7 g/dL) improves patient outcomes and reduces mortality as compared to a liberal transfusion strategy (goal Hgb >9 g/dL).

COMMENTARY

Through the early 2000s, a transfusion threshold of 10 g/dL was recommended for patients with acute UGIB, largely because this group was excluded from major trials showing benefit to restrictive transfusion. This trial focused specifically on patients with UGIB and was the first to demonstrate a mortality benefit associated with a restrictive transfusion strategy, with a number needed to treat to save a life of only 25 patients. Importantly, a restrictive approach may not be generalizable to UGIB patients with massive exsanguination, symptomatic cardiovascular disease, or not undergoing urgent endoscopy. Nonetheless, this study furnished crucial data supporting a restrictive transfusion strategy in most cases of acute UGIB.

Question

Should most patients with acute UGIB and Hgb >7 g/dL be transfused?

Answer

No, restrictive transfusion decreases mortality, complications, and rebleeding as compared to a liberal approach.

CHAPTER 39

PPI BEFORE ENDOSCOPY IN UGIB

Nadim Mahmud

Omeprazole Before Endoscopy in Patients With Gastrointestinal Bleeding
Lau JY, Leung WK, Wu JCY, et al. *N Engl J Med*. 2007;356(16):1631–1640

BACKGROUND

In patients with acute upper gastrointestinal bleeding (UGIB), proton pump inhibitors (PPIs) promote platelet aggregation and clot formation by neutralizing gastric pH. At the time of this article, high-dose PPI after endoscopic therapy had been shown to reduce recurrent bleeding and improve clinical outcomes in these patients. However, there were no clear data to support PPI use prior to endoscopic therapy.

OBJECTIVES

To determine if high-dose PPI prior to endoscopy reduced the need for endoscopic therapy and improved clinical outcomes in patients with UGIB.

METHODS

Randomized, double-blind, placebo-controlled trial in a Chinese hospital from 2004 to 2005.

Patients

638 patients presenting with UGIB. Exclusion criteria included long-term aspirin therapy for cardiovascular protection, age <18, and refractory hypotensive shock requiring urgent endoscopy.

Interventions

Omeprazole (80 mg intravenous bolus and 8 mg/hr infusion) versus an identical-appearing placebo. In both groups, endoscopy was performed the following morning, with 72 hours of open-label intravenous omeprazole given to those receiving endoscopic ulcer therapy.

Outcomes

The primary outcome was the need for endoscopic therapy during initial endoscopy. Secondary outcomes included signs of bleeding during endoscopy, need for transfusion, need for urgent endoscopy or emergency surgery for hemostasis, duration of hospital stay, and rates of recurrent bleeding and death within 30 days.

KEY RESULTS

- Fewer patients required endoscopic therapy in the omeprazole group (19.1% vs. 28.4%, RR 0.67, 95% CI 0.51–0.90, $p = 0.007$).
- During endoscopy among those with ulcers, the omeprazole group had fewer actively bleeding (6.4% vs. 14.7%, $p = 0.01$) and more clean-based (64.2% vs. 47.4%, $p = 0.001$) ulcers.
- Median length of stay was shorter in the omeprazole group ($p = 0.003$) but there were otherwise no differences in mean number of blood transfusions ($p = 0.12$), need for urgent endoscopy ($p = 0.79$) or emergency surgery ($p = 1.00$), recurrent bleeding ($p = 0.49$), or death ($p = 0.78$).

STUDY CONCLUSIONS

In patients with acute UGIB, early intravenous omeprazole therapy reduced the number of actively bleeding ulcers on endoscopy and decreased the need for endoscopic therapy.

COMMENTARY

This trial suggested a compelling physiologic rationale for benefit in a common and highly morbid condition – namely that PPI therapy can reduce active bleeding and the need for endoscopic therapy, presumably by accelerating hemostasis. The major caveats of this study are its single-center design, homogenous patient group, and – most importantly – the lack of a mortality benefit. Indeed, the 2012 American College of Gastroenterology bleeding peptic ulcer guidelines recognize these shortcomings, stating that "pre-endoscopic PPI may be considered to decrease the need for endoscopic therapy but does not improve clinical outcomes." Of note, the study authors later released a cost–benefit analysis demonstrating a reduction in hospital cost associated with pre-endoscopic PPI therapy.[1] Though the current ideal dose, regimen, and route of delivery are controversial and evolving, PPI therapy is very frequently employed before endoscopy in cases of acute UGIB.

Question

Is it reasonable to start a PPI in most patients presenting with an acute UGIB?

Answer

Yes, pre-endoscopic PPI therapy decreases signs of endoscopic bleeding and reduces the need for endoscopic therapy in patients admitted for acute UGIB, although it does not affect mortality.

References

1. Tsoi KK, Lau JY, Sung JJ. Cost-effectiveness analysis of high-dose omeprazole infusion before endoscopy for patients with upper-GI bleeding. *Gastrointest Endosc.* 2008;67(7):1056–1063.

CHAPTER 40

ALBUMIN IN SBP

Ersilia M. DeFilippis

Effect of Intravenous Albumin on Renal Impairment and Mortality in Patients With Cirrhosis and Spontaneous Bacterial Peritonitis

Sort P, Navasa M, Arroyo V, et al. *N Engl J Med*. 1999;341(6):403–409

BACKGROUND

One-third of cirrhotic patients with spontaneous bacterial peritonitis (SBP) develop renal impairment, a complication which predicts increased in-hospital mortality. Patients with SBP have splanchnic vasodilation leading to renin-induced vasoconstriction and decreased renal perfusion. Albumin increases oncotic pressure, thereby preventing the third-spacing which can occur with crystalloid fluids. However, at the time of this study, there were no high quality data evaluating the effect of albumin in SBP.

OBJECTIVES

To determine whether treatment with intravenous albumin prevents renal impairment and reduces mortality in patients with SBP.

METHODS

Randomized controlled, open-label trial at 7 Spanish centers between 1995 and 1997.

Patients

126 patients. Inclusion criteria included cirrhosis with SBP as diagnosed by >250 neutrophils in the ascitic fluid, and age between 18 and 80 years. Exclusion criteria included suspicion of secondary peritonitis, treatment with antibiotics within the preceding week (with the exception of prophylactic norfloxacin), presence of other infections, shock, gastrointestinal bleeding, hepatic encephalopathy, organic nephropathy, creatinine >3 mg/dL, or potential causes of dehydration including diarrhea within 1 week prior.

Intervention

Albumin (1.5 g/kg on day 1 and 1 g/kg on day 3) versus no intervention (control). All patients received renally dosed cefotaxime.

Outcomes

The primary outcome was development of renal impairment, defined as a nonreversible increase of either blood urea nitrogen (BUN) or serum creatinine by >50% during the hospitalization. In patients without pre-existing renal disease, the definition additionally required a BUN >30 mg/dL or creatinine >1.5 mg/dL. Other outcomes included mortality both in-hospital and at 3 months.

KEY RESULTS

- Renal impairment occurred in 6/63 (10%) of the albumin group compared to 21/63 (33%) of the control group ($p = 0.002$).
- In-hospital death occurred in 6/63 (10%) of the albumin group compared to 18/63 (29%) of the control group ($p = 0.01$).
- Death at 3 months occurred in 14/63 (22%) of the albumin group and in 26/63 (41%) of the control group ($p = 0.03$).
- Other predictors of mortality included BUN ≥30 mg/dL, bilirubin ≥4 mg/dL, and elevated prothrombin time at baseline.

STUDY CONCLUSIONS

Administration of albumin prevents renal impairment and reduces mortality in cirrhotic patients with SBP.

COMMENTARY

This study confirmed that renal failure in cirrhotic patients with SBP is an indicator of poor prognosis and increased mortality. Two limitations deserve mention. First, although the study was randomized, it was nonblinded. Second, posttreatment markers of intravascular volume depletion including renin and sodium were significantly different between the two groups, which the authors attribute to effective resuscitation with albumin, although fluid resuscitation in the cefotaxime-alone group was inadequately documented. A follow-up study examined a "restricted use" approach to administration of albumin in patients with SBP. Only patients with bilirubin >4 mg/dL or creatinine >1 mg/dL were treated with albumin. Renal impairment did not develop in the low-risk patients without these laboratory abnormalities. These 2 studies informed the American Association for the Study of Liver Diseases 2012 ascites guidelines, which recommend that patients with SBP as well as a serum creatinine >1 mg/dL, BUN >30 mg/dL, or total bilirubin >4 mg/dL receive albumin therapy within 6 hours of detection and on day 3.

Question

Should selected patients with SBP receive albumin?

Answer

Yes, treatment with albumin reduces renal impairment and mortality in many patients with cirrhosis and SBP. This benefit may be primarily in those with elevated creatinine, BUN, or total bilirubin.

References

1. Sigal SH, Stanca CM, Fernandez J, Arroyo V, Navasa M. Restricted use of albumin for spontaneous bacterial peritonitis. *Gut.* 2007;56: 597–599.

CHAPTER 41

10-YEAR INTERVAL FOR SCREENING COLONOSCOPY

Nadim Mahmud

Risk of Developing Colorectal Cancer Following a Negative Colonoscopy Examination: Evidence for a 10-Year Interval Between Colonoscopies

Singh H, Turner D, Xue L, Targownik LE, Bernstein CN. *JAMA.* 2006;295(20):2366–2373

BACKGROUND

Colonoscopy is a leading modality for colorectal cancer (CRC) screening. However, prior to this study, the recommended 10-year screening interval was based primarily on estimates of adenoma to carcinoma transformation time, and there was no evidence of durable decreased CRC risk after negative colonoscopy.

OBJECTIVES

To ascertain the degree and duration of decreased CRC risk in an average-risk population following negative colonoscopy.

METHODS

Population-based retrospective study of provincial government universal health insurance database in Manitoba, Canada between 1989 and 2003.

Patients

35,975 patients with negative index colonoscopies, defined as those without polypectomy or biopsy. Exclusion criteria included previous CRC or colorectal resection, inflammatory bowel disease, and lower endoscopy in the 5 years prior to the index procedure.

Outcomes

The primary outcome was incidence rate of CRC in the cohort, with person-years at risk accruing until CRC diagnosis, death, or migration from Manitoba. These data were used to create standardized incidence ratios (SIRs), calculated as the observed incidence rate of CRC in the study cohort divided by the expected incidence rate in the general provincial population, adjusted for age, sex, and calendar year. CRCs were characterized as right or left sided for analysis.

KEY RESULTS

- CRC risk remained reduced through 10 years of observation after negative colonoscopy, with specific SIRs as follows: 0.69 at 6 months (95% CI 0.59–0.81), 0.66 at 1 year (95% CI 0.56–0.78), 0.59 at 2 years (95% CI 0.48–0.72), 0.55 at 5 years (95% CI 0.41–0.73), and 0.28 at 10 years (95% CI 0.09–0.65).

STUDY CONCLUSIONS

Negative colonoscopy is associated with a reduced CRC risk for at least 10 years.

COMMENTARY

This study demonstrated that negative colonoscopy is associated with reduced CRC risk through 10 years of follow-up. There are 2 caveats to these results. First, although higher-risk patients were excluded from the study cohort, the expected CRC incidence rate in the general population was not similarly adjusted, potentially leading to overestimation of the risk reduction in the study cohort. Second, the SIRs decreased over time with early CRC risk reduction in the 30% to 40% range, a finding that might be explained by false-negative index colonoscopies resulting in a disproportionate number of CRCs early in the study period. The 10-year SIR, however, should be less affected by false-negative colonoscopies and therefore reflect the true risk reduction associated with negative index colonoscopy. Indeed, CRC risk reduction at 10 years was comparable to that observed in patients receiving colonoscopy and polypectomy.[1] As a result of this data, the 2009 American College of Gastroenterology CRC screening guidelines continue to endorse a 10-year screening interval after negative colonoscopy.

Question

Is 10 years an appropriate screening interval following negative colonoscopy for average-risk patients?

Answer

Yes, a negative colonoscopy is associated with a 70% CRC risk reduction at 10 years of follow-up.

References

1. Winawer SJ, Zauber AG, Ho MN, et al; The National Polyp Study Workgroup. Prevention of colorectal cancer by colonoscopic polypectomy. *N Engl J Med.* 1993;329(27):1977–1981.

CHAPTER 42

SAAG IN THE DIAGNOSIS OF ASCITES

Nadim Mahmud

The Serum-Ascites Albumin Gradient is Superior to the Exudate–Transudate Concept in the Differential Diagnosis of Ascites

Runyon BA, Montano AA, Akriviadis EA, Antillon MR, Irving MA, McHutchison JG. *Ann Intern Med.* 1992;117(3):215–220

BACKGROUND

The classic understanding of ascites relied on the exudate–transudate concept. In this model, inflammatory or neoplastic processes cause protein-rich exudative ascites, whereas Starling force imbalances, as seen in heart failure or cirrhosis, cause protein-poor transudates. While the ascites fluid total protein (AFTP) measurement was standard for distinguishing exudates from transudates, it led to numerous misclassifications. Noting that false exudates were often related to increased serum protein levels, the serum-ascites albumin gradient (SAAG) was proposed as an alternative metric to improve ascites characterization. The SAAG differentiates ascites etiologies based on the presence or absence of portal hypertension (PHT) rather than classification as an exudate or transudate.

OBJECTIVES

To compare the SAAG with the AFTP in differentiating etiologies of ascites.

METHODS

Prospective study between 1983 and 1989.

Patients

330 patients yielding 901 paired ascites and serum samples. Inclusion criteria were a confirmed etiology of ascites.

Interventions

Sample testing (cell count and differential, cytology, culture, and tuberculosis testing) and adjunct patient data (hepatic venous pressure gradient, biopsy, ultrasound, endoscopy, and/or postmortem findings, depending on clinical circumstance) were used to determine the etiology of ascites for each sample. Samples were further classified according to exudate or transudate, and the presence or absence of PHT. The SAAG and AFTP approaches were then applied to categorize samples, using PHT (SAAG) or exudate–transudate (AFTP).

Outcomes

The primary outcome was accuracy of ascites classification, calculated as the sum of true-positive and true-negative results divided by the total number of samples. Secondary outcomes included the effect of diuresis on the SAAG and AFTP.

KEY RESULTS

- The SAAG more accurately classified ascites (96.7%) compared to the AFTP (55.6%).
- The SAAG was unaffected by diuresis (18.1–18.3 g/L, p = NS), whereas the AFTP increased significantly (9.3–15.8 g/L, p < 0.0001).

STUDY CONCLUSIONS

In patients with various forms of ascites, the SAAG is superior to the AFTP in classifying ascites etiology.

COMMENTARY

The AFTP frequently misclassified the etiology of ascites by using the exudate–transudate distinction. The SAAG emerged as a more physiologic alternative affected principally by portal pressures. Although previously evaluated, this study was the first to use the SAAG to categorize ascites based on the presence or absence of PHT rather than as exudates or transudates. Furthermore, it included many causes of ascites and an exhaustive diagnostic workup to confirm true etiologies. The authors showed that the SAAG was far more accurate than the AFTP in classifying ascites. Based on this work, the 2012 American Association for the Study of Liver Diseases guidelines on ascites due to cirrhosis recommend a SAAG-based PHT classification system, effectively replacing the exudate–transudate concept in the workup of ascitic fluid.

Question

Is the SAAG useful in discriminating the etiology of ascites?

Answer

Yes, the SAAG is highly accurate in classifying ascites as PHT related or not, and is more effective than the AFTP and the exudate–transudate approach.

CHAPTER 43

RIFAXIMIN IN HEPATIC ENCEPHALOPATHY

Ersilia M. DeFilippis

Rifaximin Treatment in Hepatic Encephalopathy

Bass NM, Mullen KD, Sanyal A, et al. *N Engl J Med*. 2010;362(12):1071–1081

BACKGROUND

At the time of this study, the standard of care to prevent hepatic encephalopathy (HE) was treatment with lactulose. However, lactulose has an overly sweet taste and can cause gastrointestinal distress, leading to poor adherence. Rifaximin is a well-tolerated, non-toxic, and minimally absorbed oral antibiotic that concentrates in the gastrointestinal tract and, for these reasons, was thought to be more amenable to long-term use. Rifaximin had been shown to be superior to nonabsorbable disaccharides like lactulose in the treatment of acute HE. However, its efficacy as preventative therapy had not been established.

OBJECTIVES

To assess the efficacy of rifaximin in the prevention of HE.

METHODS

Randomized, double-blind, placebo-controlled trial at 70 centers across North America and Russia from 2005 to 2008.

Patients

299 patients. Inclusion criteria included ≥2 episodes of cirrhosis-associated HE during the previous 6 months, remission of HE at enrollment, age ≥18 years, and model for end-stage liver disease (MELD) score ≤25. Exclusion criteria included expectation of liver transplantation within 1 month or presence of conditions known to precipitate HE (e.g., transjugular intrahepatic portosystemic shunt or gastrointestinal hemorrhage requiring transfusion).

Intervention

Oral rifaximin (550 mg twice daily) versus placebo for 6 months or until discontinuation of study drug due to breakthrough episode of HE.

Outcomes

The primary outcome was time to first breakthrough episode of HE. Major secondary outcomes included time to first hospitalization for HE or complicated by HE.

KEY RESULTS

- Over a 6-month period, 31/140 (22.1%) in the rifaximin group had breakthrough HE episodes compared to 73/159 (45.9%) in the placebo group (HR 0.42, 95% CI 0.28–0.64, $p < 0.001$).
- Hospitalization for HE or complicated by HE occurred in 19/140 (13.6%) of the rifaximin group compared to 36/159 (22.6%) of the placebo group (HR 0.50, 95% CI 0.29–0.87, $p = 0.01$).
- The rate of adverse events was similar in the rifaximin and placebo groups.

STUDY CONCLUSIONS

Treatment with rifaximin is protective against episodes of HE and reduces the risk of hospitalization involving HE.

COMMENTARY

These findings solidified the role for rifaximin in preventing breakthrough HE episodes (number needed to treat = 4) and hospitalization for, or complicated by, HE (number needed to treat = 11). Over 90% of patients were also on lactulose in addition to the study drug, raising the question of whether rifaximin is sufficient as monotherapy. Although study patients were at high risk for HE, as evidenced by a history of recurrent encephalopathy, patients with the highest MELD scores were excluded. The updated 2014 American Association for the Study of Liver Disease HE guidelines now include rifaximin as an effective add-on therapy to lactulose for prevention of HE recurrence.

Question

Does treatment with rifaximin reduce the risk of further episodes of HE in high-risk patients?

Answer

Yes, when combined with lactulose in patients with recent history of recurrent overt HE, rifaximin reduces the risk of breakthrough HE episodes and HE hospitalizations.

CHAPTER 44

"TOP-DOWN" THERAPY FOR CROHN DISEASE

Ersilia M. DeFilippis

Early Combined Immunosuppression or Conventional Management in Patients With Newly Diagnosed Crohn's Disease: An Open Randomized Trial

D'Haens G, Baert F, van Assche G, et al. *Lancet.* 2008;371(9613):660–667

BACKGROUND

At the time of this study, the treatment convention for Crohn disease (CD) consisted of a "step-up" approach starting with corticosteroid therapy and the addition of immuno-modulators for steroid-refractory or steroid-dependent patients. Biologic agents, such as tumor necrosis factor (TNF) inhibitors, were reserved for patients who had failed both of these therapies. A "top-down" approach, which included early combination immunosuppression with a TNF inhibitor, had been shown to be effective in rheuma-toid arthritis. However, a top-down strategy had not been applied to CD.

OBJECTIVES

To compare the effectiveness of early combined immunosuppression with conventional management in CD patients.

METHODS

Randomized, open-label trial at 18 European centers between 2001 and 2004.

Patients

133 patients with active CD. Inclusion criteria included age 16 to 75 years and CD diagnosis within the past 4 years without any previous treatment with steroids, antime-tabolites, or biologic agents. Exclusion criteria included symptomatic stenosis, strictures, chronic infection (including positive tuberculin test), malignancy, positive stool culture, and immediate need for surgery.

Interventions

Early combined immunosuppression versus conventional therapy. The early combined immunosuppression group received infliximab (5 mg/kg at weeks 0, 2, and 6) and an antimetabolite (azathioprine, or methotrexate if intolerant to azathioprine), with rescue therapy of additional infliximab or methylprednisolone while continuing the antime-tabolite. The conventional therapy group received 10 weeks of tapered methylpredniso-lone or budesonide, with rescue therapy of methylprednisolone and azathioprine; those who remained symptomatic after 16 weeks of azathioprine started infliximab. Patients were followed for 104 weeks.

Outcomes

The 2 primary outcomes were remission, without corticosteroids and without bowel resection, at 26 and 52 weeks. Secondary outcomes included time to relapse after successful induction and endoscopic severity scores.

KEY RESULTS

- At 26 weeks, a higher proportion of the combined immunosuppression group was in remission compared to those in the conventional therapy group (60.0% vs. 35.9%, $p = 0.0062$). The difference persisted at 52 weeks (61.5% vs. 42.2%, $p = 0.0278$).
- The frequency of longer-term remission did not differ between the 2 groups ($p = 0.797$ at 78 weeks, $p = 0.431$ at 104 weeks).
- Median time to relapse after successful induction was longer for those in the early combined immunosuppression group (329 days vs. 174.5 days, $p = 0.031$).
- At week 104, more of the early combined immunosuppression group was ulcer free (19/26, 73.1% vs. 7/23, 30.4%, $p = 0.0028$).

STUDY CONCLUSIONS

The use of early combined immunosuppression in CD resulted in earlier and more frequent remission than treatment according to existing guidelines.

COMMENTARY

This pivotal study demonstrated that upfront combination immunosuppression inclusive of a TNF inhibitor resulted in higher rates of remission than conventional therapy. Caveats included small sample size, unblinded design, and concurrent evolution of clinical practice during the study period away from intermittent infliximab regimens used in the trial toward continuous dosing. Nonetheless, study findings were affirmed in the SONIC study,[1] which showed that infliximab, alone or in combination with azathioprine, was superior to azathioprine alone. Together, these results informed the 2013 American Gastroenterological Association guidelines on medical management of CD, which recommend a top-down approach for patients with moderate to severe CD consisting of anti-TNF and thiopurine combination therapy.

Question

Is early combined immunosuppression with a top-down approach reasonable in active CD?

Answer

Yes, treatment with combined immunosuppression early in the course of active CD is more likely to induce clinical remission than conventional therapy.

References

1. Colombel JF, Sandborn WJ, Reinisch W, et al. Infliximab, azathioprine, or combination therapy for Crohn's Disease. *N Engl J Med.* 2010;362(15):1383–1395.

HEMATOLOGY

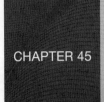

PLASMA EXCHANGE IN THROMBOTIC THROMBOCYTOPENIC PURPURA

CHAPTER 45

Gabriel B. Loeb

Comparison of Plasma Exchange with Plasma Infusion in the Treatment of Thrombotic Thrombocytopenic Purpura.

Rock GA, Shumak KH, Buskard NA, et al. *N Engl J Med*. 1991;325(6):393–397

BACKGROUND
Untreated thrombotic thrombocytopenic purpura (TTP) has a 90% mortality rate. At the time of this trial, several case studies had shown treatment with plasma was effective; however, no study had directly compared delivery of plasma through simple infusion to exchange transfusion.

OBJECTIVE
To determine whether plasma exchange or plasma infusion is a more effective treatment for TTP.

METHODS
Randomized, controlled, open-label trial in 27 Canadian hospitals from 1982 to 1989.

Patients
102 patients. Inclusion criteria included TTP (defined by platelet count <100,000/μL and red-cell fragmentation on peripheral smear without identifiable alternative etiology of thrombocytopenia or microangiopathic hemolytic anemia). Exclusion criteria included heart failure or anuria that would prevent plasma infusion.

Interventions
Plasma exchange with fresh-frozen plasma (FFP) ≥7 times over the first 9 days versus daily FFP infusions. All patients received dipyridamole (400 mg daily) and aspirin (325 mg daily). Crossover from infusion to exchange was permitted in the event of treatment failure.

Outcomes
The outcomes included 6-month survival, complete response (CR) at 7 days and 6 months (defined as platelet count >150,000/μL for 2 consecutive days with stable neurologic status), and adverse events.

KEY RESULTS

- 6-month survival was higher in the exchange arm (78% vs. 63%, $p = 0.036$). Of the 51 patients in the infusion arm, 20 received plasma infusion alone (50% survival) and 31 crossed over to plasma exchange (71% survival).
- At 7 days, the rate of CR was higher in the exchange arm (47% vs. 25%, $p = 0.025$). At 6 months, the CR rates were 78% in the exchange arm and 49% in the infusion arm.
- 4 patients in each group had seizures during treatment. 1 patient receiving plasma exchange died of a gastrointestinal bleed. 41 patients had nausea and 34 had hypotension; breakdown by study arm was not reported.

STUDY CONCLUSIONS

Plasma exchange leads to better response rates and overall survival than plasma infusion for patients with TTP.

COMMENTARY

This trial, along with a large case series published simultaneously,[1] helped establish plasma exchange as the gold-standard therapy for TTP. Given the low incidence of TTP, the study was particularly remarkable for its size, enrolling nearly all the cases of TTP occurring in Canada over a 7-year period. Caveats include the lack of classification of TTP cases by the underlying cause (e.g., idiopathic or related to pregnancy, medication, pancreatitis, or infection), which influences management and prognosis. Additionally, all patients in the study received aspirin and dipyridamole, which are no longer routinely used, but not glucocorticoids, which are now an important part of initial therapy. Largely due to this study, the 2012 British Committee for Standards in Hematology TTP guidelines recommend plasma exchange and glucocorticoids as initial therapy for TTP.

Question

Should patients receive plasma exchange rather than plasma infusion for treatment of TTP?

Answer

Yes, plasma exchange is the treatment of choice for TTP.

References

1. Bell WR, Braine HG, Ness PM, Kickler TS. Improved survival in thrombotic thrombocytopenic purpura-hemolytic uremic syndrome. Clinical experience in 108 patients. *N Engl J Med.* 1991;325(6):398–403.

CHAPTER 46

NATURAL HISTORY AND PROGNOSIS OF MGUS

Ersilia M. DeFilippis

A Long-Term Study of Prognosis in Monoclonal Gammopathy of Undetermined Significance

Kyle RA, Therneau TM, Rajkumar SV, et al. *N Engl J Med*. 2002;346(8):564–569

BACKGROUND

Patients over the age of 50 are commonly affected by monoclonal gammopathy of undetermined significance (MGUS). Previous investigations had suggested that malignant transformation could occur in up to 20% of patients over 5 to 10 years. However, these studies had relatively small sample sizes, short follow-up time, or possible referral bias. As a result, it was unknown which factors predicted progression from MGUS to multiple myeloma or related blood disorders.

OBJECTIVES

To determine the prognosis and predictors of outcomes in a large geographic cohort of patients with MGUS.

METHODS

Retrospective cohort study of medical records and vital status from 1 American center from 1960 to 1994.

Patients

1,384 MGUS patients from southern Minnesota.

Intervention

The MGUS cohort was followed for a median of 15.4 years, over which time risk factors for progression to malignant disease were assessed. Survival rates were compared between the MGUS cohort and an age- and sex-matched control population.

Outcomes

Primary outcome was progression to multiple myeloma or other B-cell or lymphoid cancer (lymphoma with IgM serum monoclonal protein, primary amyloidosis, macroglobulinemia, chronic lymphocytic leukemia, or plasmacytoma). Secondary outcomes included death from plasma cell disorders or other causes. Predictors of progression were also assessed.

KEY RESULTS

- The median age of MGUS diagnosis was 72 years, and MGUS progressed to multiple myeloma or other B-cell or lymphoid cancer at a rate of 1% per year.
- Among the MGUS cohort, the risk of malignant progression increased with increasing baseline monoclonal protein concentration ($p < 0.001$).
- Compared to those with IgG monoclonal protein, MGUS patients with IgM or IgA monoclonal protein had an increased risk of malignant progression ($p = 0.001$).
- Among the MGUS cohort, death from other causes (53%) was more common than death from plasma cell disorders (6%) at 10 years.
- MGUS patients had shorter median survival than age- and sex-matched controls (8.1 years vs. 11.8 years, $p < 0.001$).
- Median survival was shorter in the MGUS cohort than age- and sex-matched controls (8.1 years vs. 11.8 years, $p < 0.001$).

STUDY CONCLUSIONS

Patients with MGUS are at increased risk for progression to multiple myeloma or a related plasma cell cancer, as well as death.

COMMENTARY

This pivotal study helped to establish a risk stratification model for patients with MGUS and guide future monitoring and management efforts. The strengths of this study include its large population and prolonged follow-up. It updated and added precision and greater accuracy to previous estimates of the rate of transformation, while also providing crucial prognostic information. Informed by this investigation, the 2010 International Myeloma Working Group MGUS and smoldering myeloma monitoring and management guidelines recommend that all patients are risk stratified at the time of MGUS diagnosis. The 3 most significant risk factors include an abnormal free light chain ratio, nonimmunoglobulin G MGUS, and high serum M protein level.

Question

Does MGUS increase the risk of progression to multiple myeloma and other plasma cell related disorders?

Answer

Yes, MGUS increases the risk of progression to multiple myeloma and other plasma cell disorders. The initial concentration of serum monoclonal protein and the nature of the immunoglobulin are important risk factors.

CHAPTER 47

THE *JAK2* MUTATION IN MYELOPROLIFERATIVE NEOPLASMS

Gabriel B. Loeb

A Unique Clonal *JAK2* Mutation Leading to Constitutive Signalling Causes Polycythaemia Vera

James C, Ugo V, Le Couédic JP, et al. *Nature*. 2005;434(7037):1144–1148

BACKGROUND

At the time of this report, there were no known molecular drivers of polycythemia vera (PCV), essential thrombocytosis (ET), or primary myelofibrosis (PMF). The identification of a recurrent driver mutation was important for understanding the molecular pathways involved in these myeloproliferative neoplasms (MPNs), improving disease classification → facilitating diagnosis, and aiding in the development of targeted therapies.

OBJECTIVES

To determine the molecular driver of PCV.

METHODS

A short interfering RNA (siRNA) against *JAK2* was used in a cell line and cells derived from patient samples to ascertain *JAK2*'s role in erythroid development. Targeted sequencing of the *JAK2* gene identified mutations in patients with MPNs. Retroviral overexpression of mutant *JAK2* in cell lines and mouse bone marrow was used to examine the mutation's effect on signaling, cell growth, and hematopoiesis.

Patients

128 patients who underwent genetic sequencing (The *JAK2* exons and intron–exon junctions were initially sequenced in 3 PCV patients and 2 controls. An exon containing a mutation identified in the original cohort was then sequenced in 45 PCV patients, 7 PMF patients, 21 ET patients, 35 patients with secondary erythrocytosis, and 15 controls). PCV patients had elevated red cell mass, no known cause of secondary erythrocytosis, endogenous erythroid colony formation, and one of the following: splenomegaly, neutrophilia, thrombocytosis, or a clonal marker.

KEY RESULTS

- The *JAK2* valine to phenylalanine mutation at amino acid 617 (V617F) was found in 40/45 patients with PCV, 3/7 with PMF, 9/21 with ET, 0/15 controls, and 0/35 with secondary erythrocytosis.
- When *JAK2* V617F but not wild-type *JAK2* was transfected into interleukin-3- or erythropoietin-dependent cell lines, cytokine-independent growth and cytokine hypersensitivity were observed. *JAK2* V617F transfection also promoted enhanced

cytokine-independent phosphorylation of genes known to promote cellular proliferation.

- In bone marrow cells from about 30% of PCV patients, only the V617F allele was detected and the wild-type allele was lost.
- The average hematocrit in mice transplanted with bone marrow expressing wild-type *JAK2* was 40%, while those with bone marrow expressing V617F *JAK2* had hematocrits of 60% ($p < 0.001$).

STUDY CONCLUSIONS

The *JAK2* V617F mutation is an acquired mutation in a large proportion of PCV patients and many other patients with MPNs. This mutation leads to polycythemia through hematopoietic progenitor cytokine hypersensitivity/independence.

COMMENTARY

Although the clonal nature of MPNs was understood, the molecular drivers of their phenotypes and proliferation were unknown before this study. The *JAK2* V617F mutation it described also was subsequently reported within 1 month by 3 other groups. The mutation is present in most patients with PCV and many with ET and PMF. The ability to definitively diagnose PCV using a molecular test represents a major advance, and the presence of *JAK2* V617F or a *JAK2* exon 12 mutation is now a major criterion in the World Health Organization diagnostic criteria for PCV. *JAK2* inhibitors currently have a limited role in treatment of PCV and PMF, but clinical trials in this area are ongoing.

Question

Is a specific mutation associated with the development of PCV?

Answer

Yes, an activating mutation in *JAK2,* most commonly V617F, is present in most PCV patients and many with PMF and ET.

CHAPTER 48

IMATINIB FOR CML

Gabriel B. Loeb

Five-Year Follow-up of Patients Receiving Imatinib for Chronic Myeloid Leukemia
Druker BJ, Guilhot F, O'Brien SG, et al. *N Engl J Med*. 2006;355(23):2408–2417

BACKGROUND

By 2003, imatinib (a BCR-ABL tyrosine kinase inhibitor) had demonstrated superior response rates and lower toxicity than standard chemotherapy (cytarabine and interferon alfa) in chronic myeloid leukemia (CML).[1] However, long-term survival outcomes with imatinib therapy were unknown.

OBJECTIVE

To establish the 5-year efficacy and tolerability of imatinib for treatment-naïve patients with chronic phase CML.

METHODS

Long-term follow-up of a randomized, controlled, open-label, multicenter trial[1] from 2000 to 2006.

Patients

This study reported results from the 553 patients initially randomized to imatinib therapy out of 1,106 patients in the initial trial. Inclusion criteria included age 18 to 70 years, Philadelphia chromosome–positive CML, and no previous treatment (except for hydroxyurea or anagrelide). Exclusion criteria included extramedullary disease (other than hepatosplenomegaly), and abnormal renal or hepatic function.

Interventions

5-year analysis of patients initially randomized to receive imatinib.

Outcomes

The primary outcome was event-free survival (EFS) at 60 months (events defined as loss of hematologic or cytogenetic response or progression to accelerated phase CML or blast crisis) in the imatinib group. Secondary outcomes included overall survival (OS) at 60 months and rate of adverse events (neutropenia, thrombocytopenia, anemia, and others), and medication tolerability.

KEY RESULTS

- 60-month EFS of patients receiving imatinib as initial therapy was 83% (95% CI, 79%–87%).
- 60-month OS of patients receiving imatinib as initial therapy was 89% (95% CI, 86%–92%).

- Neutropenia was the most common severe adverse event and occurred in 14% of patients in years 1 and 2, 3% patients in years 3 and 4, and 1% after year 4.
- 5 years after the last patient was randomized, 69% of those assigned to the imatinib group continued taking this therapy versus 3% continuing initial treatment in the standard therapy group.
- The most common reasons for cessation of imatinib were unsatisfactory therapeutic effect (11%), withdrawal of consent (5%), adverse event (4%), stem-cell transplant (3%), or death (2%).

STUDY CONCLUSIONS

Continuous treatment of chronic-phase CML with imatinib is effective, well tolerated, and leads to excellent OS.

COMMENTARY

The initial phase 3 data for imatinib demonstrated superior effectiveness and tolerability relative to standard chemotherapy. This 5-year follow-up report confirmed that imatinib was well tolerated over a longer period and leads to excellent OS, durable responses, and decreasing rates of relapse and adverse events with increasing time on therapy. Importantly, individuals in accelerated phase CML or blast crisis were not enrolled in this trial and continue to have poorer outcomes with current therapies. This study helped make imatinib (now joined by second-generation BCR-ABL tyrosine kinase inhibitors dasatinib and nilotinib) the standard of care treatment for CML, and ushered in the era of molecularly targeted cancer therapy. The 2016 National Comprehensive Cancer Network guidelines recommend imatinib as one of several BCR-ABL tyrosine kinase inhibitors for initial chronic phase CML therapy.

Question

Should patients with chronic phase CML be treated with a BCR-ABL tyrosine kinase inhibitor?

Answer

Yes, BCR-ABL tyrosine kinase inhibitors such as imatinib are well tolerated and lead to durable responses and excellent survival.

References

1. O'Brien SG, Guilhot F, Larson RA, et al. Imatinib compared with interferon and low-dose cytarabine for newly diagnosed chronic-phase chronic myeloid leukemia. *N Engl J Med.* 2003;348(11):994–1004.

CHAPTER 49

R-CHOP FOR DIFFUSE LARGE B-CELL LYMPHOMA: THE GELA TRIAL

Daniel O'Neil ■ Luis Ticona

CHOP Chemotherapy Plus Rituximab Compared With CHOP Alone in Elderly Patients With Diffuse Large-B-cell Lymphoma

Coiffier B, Lepage E, Brière J, et al. *N Engl J Med.* 2002;346(4):235–242

BACKGROUND

At the time of this study, cyclophosphamide, doxorubicin, vincristine, and prednisone (CHOP) chemotherapy was standard of care for diffuse large B-cell lymphoma (DLBCL), one of the most common types of lymphoma. Phase 2 studies had shown that rituximab, a monoclonal antibody targeting B lymphocytes and the first to be FDA approved for cancer treatment, was promising and safe in relapsed or refractory disease. However, no randomized, head-to-head comparisons between CHOP and CHOP plus rituximab (R-CHOP) existed.

OBJECTIVES

To compare R-CHOP versus CHOP as the initial treatment of elderly patients with DLBCL.

METHODS

Randomized, controlled study at 86 centers in 3 European countries between 1998 and 2000.

Patients

398 patients. Inclusion criteria included age 60 to 80 years and a diagnosis of stage II to IV DLBCL with good-to-fair performance status (Eastern Cooperative Oncology Group score 0–2). Exclusion criteria included central nervous system involvement, active cancer, and HIV.

Interventions

R-CHOP versus CHOP. Both arms received 8 cycles of therapy, with dose reductions for cytopenias. A planned pathologic review was conducted to confirm DLBCL diagnosis. Patients were followed for a median 24 months.

Outcomes

The primary outcome was event-free survival (EFS) rate. Events were defined as disease progression or relapse, new anticancer treatment, or death from any cause. Secondary outcomes included the rates of overall survival (OS), complete response (disappearance of all lesions and of radiologic or biologic abnormalities and the absence of new lesions), and unconfirmed complete response (complete response with persistence of some radiologic abnormalities that regressed in size by ≥75%). Severe adverse events included infection, cardiac events, and toxicity.

KEY RESULTS

- The probability of EFS (57% vs. 39%, $p = 0.002$) and OS (71% vs. 59%, $p = 0.007$) was higher in the R-CHOP group.
- The rate of complete response or unconfirmed complete response was higher in patients treated with R-CHOP (76% vs. 63%, $p = 0.005$).
- The rate of infection was similar in both groups (65% vs. 65%, no p value reported), as was that of severe cardiac toxicity (8% vs. 8%, no p value reported).
- Severe rituximab infusion reactions were noted in 9% of the R-CHOP group (mostly respiratory symptoms, chills, fever, and hypotension). These symptoms resolved in all cases with slowing or cessation of the infusion and did not limit receipt of future R-CHOP cycles.

STUDY CONCLUSIONS

R-CHOP improves EFS and OS among patients aged 60 to 80 years.

COMMENTARY

The addition of rituximab to the standard treatment of DLBCL represented the first significant improvement over CHOP chemotherapy in decades. Caveats include discovery during pathologic review that 10% to 15% of patients were incorrectly diagnosed with DLBCL. Both a longer-term analysis of the GELA cohort at 7 years and RICOVER-60, a trial of patients >60 years old with aggressive disease,[1] confirmed the results of this study, demonstrating persistent improvement in OS. Additional work showed improved 3-year survival rates with the addition of rituximab to CHOP-like therapy in patients 18 to 60 years of age. As a result of this collective evidence, the 2014 National Comprehensive Cancer Network guidelines recommend R-CHOP as first-line therapy for DLBCL for patients with early and advanced disease, excluding those with advanced cardiac disease.

Question

Should R-CHOP be considered as a first-line treatment for the majority of patients with DLBCL?

Answer

Yes, R-CHOP leads to improved survival over CHOP alone.

References

1. Pfreundschuh M, Schubert J, Ziepert M, et al. Six versus eight cycles of bi-weekly CHOP-14 with or without rituximab in elderly patients with aggressive CD20+ B-cell lymphomas: A randomised controlled trial (RICOVER-60). *Lancet Oncol.* 2008;9(2):105–116.

CHAPTER 50

HiDAC AS CONSOLIDATION THERAPY FOR AML

Viswatej Avutu ■ Luis Ticona

Intensive Postremission Chemotherapy in Adults With Acute Myeloid Leukemia. Mayer RJ, Davis RB, Schiffer CA, et al. *N Engl J Med*. 1994;331(14):896–903

BACKGROUND

Before this study, there was significant variation in approaches to consolidation chemotherapy among acute myelogenous leukemia (AML) patients who attained complete remission after induction chemotherapy. Some received a second round of induction while others underwent consolidation using varying doses of cytarabine or maintenance therapy using other agents. Though a small, randomized trial had suggested that high dose cytarabine (HiDAC) consolidation could help maintain remission, definitive assessment of this approach was lacking.

OBJECTIVES

To compare the effect of different cytarabine consolidation regimens on the duration of complete remission in AML patients in their first remission.

METHODS

Randomized, controlled trial in 28 North American centers between 1985 and 1990.

Patients

596 patients who had achieved remission with standard induction chemotherapy. Inclusion criteria included age ≥16 years with primary, untreated AML. Exclusion criteria included a history of myelodysplasia, other hematologic cancers, liver disease or alcohol abuse, uncontrolled infection, or previous radiation or cytotoxic chemotherapy.

Interventions

Standard (100 mg/m^2) versus intermediate (400 mg/m^2) versus high (3 g/m^2 twice daily) dose cytarabine. All patients were scheduled to receive 4 courses followed by 4 monthly treatments of cytarabine and daunorubicin.

Outcomes

The primary outcome was disease-free survival (DFS) at 4 years stratified by age (<40, 40 to 60, >60 years). Secondary outcomes included 4-year survival and toxicity (including treatment courses requiring hospitalizations and serious CNS toxicity).

KEY RESULTS

- DFS at 4 years varied by age (32% vs. 29% vs. 14% in patients aged <40, 40 to 60, and >60 years, respectively, $p < 0.001$).
- With respect to DFS, age-adjusted HRs were lower for the intermediate (0.75, 95% CI 0.60–0.94) and high (0.67, 95% CI 0.53–0.86) dose groups compared to the standard dose group.
- With respect to survival, age-adjusted HRs were lower for the intermediate (0.78, 95% CI 0.61–1.00) and high (0.74, 95% CI 0.57–0.96) dose groups compared to the standard dose group. For those ≤60 years old, survival rates varied with increasing cytarabine doses (35% vs. 40% vs. 52%, $p = 0.02$).
- More patients in the high dose group required hospitalization for fever and neutropenia (71% vs. 59% and 16% in the intermediate and standard dose groups, respectively, no p value reported) and sustained serious CNS toxicity (12% vs. 0% in both intermediate and standard dose groups, no p value reported).

STUDY CONCLUSIONS

HiDAC consolidation for patients ≤60 years old is associated with improved DFS and overall survival compared to lower doses of cytarabine.

COMMENTARY

This seminal study has defined the standard regimen for cytarabine consolidation therapy. Additionally, the relatively high success rates for HiDAC in younger patients rivaled those of BMT and identified an appropriate and feasible strategy for many. Caveats include the relatively low rate of cycle completion in the HiDAC group as well as a midtrial protocol change prohibiting HiDAC for older patients. The subsequent advent of cytogenetics and molecular markers in estimating AML risk has further increased the ability to target patients who may benefit from HiDAC consolidation compared to transplantation. As a result of this trial and subsequent work, the 2015 National Comprehensive Cancer Network AML guidelines suggest HiDAC consolidation therapy as an option in patients <60 years old with "better-risk cytogenetics and/or molecular abnormalities."

Question

Is it reasonable to treat AML patients of age <60 years with better-risk disease in first complete remission with HiDAC as initial consolidation therapy?

Answer

Yes, this regimen can maintain complete remission with success rates in these specifically defined patients similar to those of BMT.

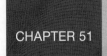

ATRA VERSUS CHEMOTHERAPY FOR ACUTE PROMYELOCYTIC LEUKEMIA

CHAPTER 51

Gabriel B. Loeb

All-*trans*-Retinoic Acid in Acute Promyelocytic Leukemia

Tallman MS, Andersen JW, Schiffer CA, et al. *N Engl J Med*. 1997;337(15):1021–1028

BACKGROUND

In the 1980s, Chinese case reports demonstrated the effectiveness of all-*trans*retinoic acid (ATRA) in acute promyelocytic leukemia (APML). Other research showed that a chromosome 15 to 17 translocation that created a retinoic acid receptor fusion protein was the causative mutation in APML and that this fusion protein was sensitive to ATRA. Although prior studies demonstrated that ATRA frequently produced complete remission in APML, definitive evidence of its effect on survival and utility as maintenance therapy was lacking.

OBJECTIVES

To compare ATRA versus chemotherapy for APML induction and ATRA versus observation for APML maintenance.

METHODS

Randomized controlled trial between 1992 and 1997.

Patients

378 patients. Inclusion criteria included APML based on bone marrow cellular morphology. Exclusion criteria included previous chemotherapy (except hydroxyurea), abnormal renal or hepatic function, and poor performance status (complete confinement to bed and/or chair).

Interventions

Oral ATRA (until complete remission or a maximum of 90 days) versus chemotherapy (daunorubicin and cytarabine). ATRA patients with leukocytosis received pretreatment with hydroxyurea and those who had unacceptable toxicity or resistant disease on ATRA could crossover to chemotherapy. All patients who achieved remission received consolidation with 2 cycles of daunorubicin and cytarabine. Patients in complete remission after induction and consolidation were randomized to 1 year of ATRA maintenance versus observation.

Outcomes

The outcomes were overall survival (OS), complete remission (CR, defined as no Auer rods and <5% blasts on bone marrow biopsy with >20% cellularity, as well as peripheral blood with greater than 1,500 neutrophils and 100,000 platelets per µL), disease-free survival (DFS, defined as complete remission without relapse or death), and toxicity.

KEY RESULTS

- OS was higher at 3 years with ATRA than with chemotherapy induction (67% vs. 50%, $p = 0.003$).
- Rate of CR was not significantly different between the ATRA and chemotherapy induction groups (72% vs. 69%, $p = 0.56$).
- There was improved DFS with ATRA relative to chemotherapy induction at 3 years (67% vs. 32%, $p < 0.001$).
- ATRA maintenance improved DFS relative to observation at 3 years (65% vs. 40%, $p < 0.001$).
- There was no significant difference in the rate of death during induction with ATRA versus chemotherapy (11% vs. 14%, $p = 0.52$).
- 26% of ATRA-induced patients developed retinoic acid syndrome.

STUDY CONCLUSIONS

ATRA induction with consolidation chemotherapy coupled with maintenance ATRA improves outcomes in APML.

COMMENTARY

This study established ATRA as a powerful first-line APML therapy. Caveats include the higher than expected relapse rate in patients who received chemotherapy alone (82% at 3 years). Subsequent trials combining ATRA with either cytotoxic therapy or arsenic trioxide have shown superior efficacy compared to ATRA alone. With current therapy, which uses these combinations for induction and consolidation, the role of maintenance therapy is unclear, particularly for patients who achieve molecular remission. The 2016 National Comprehensive Cancer Network leukemia treatment guidelines recommend ATRA, in combination with either cytotoxic therapy or arsenic trioxide, for induction and consolidation in APML.

Question

Should patients with APML receive ATRA as part of induction and consolidation therapy?

Answer

Yes, ATRA, in combination with other agents, is the treatment of choice for APML.

CHAPTER 52

BORTEZOMIB IN RELAPSED MULTIPLE MYELOMA: THE APEX TRIAL

Gabriel B. Loeb

Bortezomib or High-Dose Dexamethasone for Relapsed Multiple Myeloma

Richardson PG, Sonneveld P, Schuster MW, et al. *N Engl J Med*. 2005;352(24): 2487–2498

BACKGROUND

At the time of this study, there was no standard therapy for relapsed multiple myeloma (MM), but many regimens included high-dose dexamethasone, either alone or combined with other chemotherapeutic agents. In small studies, bortezomib, a proteasome inhibitor, had been shown to induce complete remission in relapsed/refractory MM patients. However, bortezomib had not yet been directly compared to any other therapy in a randomized trial.

OBJECTIVES

To compare bortezomib versus high-dose dexamethasone therapy in relapsed MM.

METHODS

Randomized, open-label, controlled trial at 93 centers in North America, Europe, and the Middle East from 2002 to 2003.

Patients

669 patients with MM. Inclusion criteria included progression on 1 to 3 previous treatments. Exclusion criteria included previous refractoriness to high-dose dexamethasone, previous exposure to bortezomib, poor performance status (Karnofsky performance scale ≤60), severe anemia (Hgb <7.5 g/dL), thrombocytopenia (<50,000/mm^3), neutropenia (ANC <750/mm^3), or renal failure (creatinine clearance <20 mL/min).

Interventions

Intravenous bortezomib (1.3 mg/m^2 of body surface area) versus oral dexamethasone (40 mg). All patients received bisphosphonates unless contraindicated. Patients with progression on dexamethasone were allowed to cross over to bortezomib.

Outcomes

The primary outcome was time to progression (either 25% increase in bone marrow plasma cells, 25% increase in serum or urine monoclonal immunoglobulin [M protein], new or increased bone lesions or plasmacytomas, or new hypercalcemia). Secondary outcomes included rate of response (reduction in serum M protein by 50% and urine M protein by 90%) and 1-year overall survival (OS).

KEY RESULTS

- The bortezomib group had an improved median time to progression (6.22 months vs. 3.49 months, $p < 0.001$) and response rate (38% vs. 18%, $p < 0.001$).
- Patients receiving bortezomib had superior OS at 1 year (80% vs. 66%, $p = 0.003$); 44% of patients in the dexamethasone group received bortezomib after disease progression.
- 37% of patients in the bortezomib group had adverse events requiring treatment discontinuation, compared to 29% in the dexamethasone group. Severe adverse events that were more common in the bortezomib group included thrombocytopenia (29%), neutropenia (15%), peripheral neuropathy (8%), and diarrhea (7%).

STUDY CONCLUSIONS

Bortezomib improves survival and time to progression compared to high-dose dexamethasone in relapsed MM.

COMMENTARY

APEX definitively established bortezomib as an effective therapy for relapsed MM. Caveats include the use of dexamethasone in the comparison arm despite previous glucocorticoid therapy in 98% of patients in the trial, which was neither surprising nor avoidable given the limited treatment options available to this heavily pretreated group of patients. Additionally, APEX likely underestimated bortezomib's survival benefit relative to dexamethasone due to the high treatment crossover rate. Although APEX was limited to relapsed disease, subsequent studies have established combination regimens including bortezomib and steroids such as dexamethasone as front-line myeloma therapy in both transplant-eligible and ineligible patients. The 2016 National Comprehensive Cancer Network (NCCN) MM guidelines recommend multiple bortezomib–containing regimens as induction and salvage therapy.

Question

Should bortezomib be used to treat patients with MM?

Answer

Yes, bortezomib is superior to high-dose dexamethasone for both induction and relapsed disease, and combinations including bortezomib and dexamethasone are often the treatment of choice.

CHAPTER 53

OPTIMAL THERAPY AFTER FIRST COMPLETE REMISSION IN AML

Viswatej Avutu

Chemotherapy Compared With Autologous or Allogeneic Bone Marrow Transplantation in the Management of Acute Myeloid Leukemia in First Remission

Cassileth PA, Harrington DP, Appelbaum FR, et al. *N Engl J Med.* 1998;339(23): 1649–1656

BACKGROUND

Prior to this study, several trials showed improved long-term outcomes with allogeneic bone marrow transplantation (BMT) in acute myelogenous leukemia (AML) after first complete remission (CR). Whether this strategy was superior to postremission treatment with either high-intensity chemotherapy or autologous BMT was unknown.

OBJECTIVES

To identify the optimal therapeutic option in adults with AML in first CR.

METHODS

Two linked studies – a randomized, open-label, controlled trial and an additional prospective cohort arm – between 1990 and 1995.

Patients

346 patients. Inclusion criteria included age 16 to 55 years and untreated AML. Exclusion criteria included lack of CR after 2 cycles of induction, contraindication to BMT, or severe organ impairment (renal, hepatic, or cardiac).

Interventions

Post-CR allogeneic BMT if genotypically or phenotypically HLA-matched, or single-antigen–mismatched donor available. If no allogeneic donor was available, post-CR patients were randomized to autologous BMT versus high-dose cytarabine (HDAC). All patients received a similar induction regimen (idarubicin and cytarabine). All transplant patients received the same preparative regimen (busulfan and cyclophosphamide).

Outcomes

The primary outcomes were disease-free survival (DFS, defined as lack of relapse or death from any cause after CR was achieved) and overall survival (OS), at 4 years.

KEY RESULTS

- DFS was not statistically significantly different among the 3 groups (35% HDAC, 35% autologous BMT, and 43% allogeneic BMT, p not reported). Among those without potential donors, there was no difference in DFS between HDAC and autologous BMT ($p = 0.77$).
- OS was greater following HDAC compared to autologous or allogeneic BMT (52% HDAC, 43% autologous BMT, and 46% allogeneic BMT; HDAC vs. autologous BMT, $p = 0.05$, and HDAC vs. allogeneic BMT, $p = 0.04$).
- Relapse was more common with HDAC compared to autologous or allogeneic BMT (61% HDAC vs. 48% autologous BMT vs. 29% allogeneic BMT, no p value reported).

STUDY CONCLUSIONS

While the 3 therapies studied result in similar DFS, HDAC is associated with higher rates of relapse but provides improved OS compared to autologous BMT in first CR in adults with AML. Allogeneic BMT is associated with less relapse but also less OS in adults with AML.

COMMENTARY

This trial was one of the earliest head-to-head comparisons of the primary AML therapies. It showed both the benefit of allogeneic BMT – those who survived it appeared to have a lower risk of relapse – and the increased risk for treatment-related mortality. The advent of cytogenetic markers and other molecular prognostication tools have allowed for the identification of high-risk patients whose elevated predicted mortality justifies an allogeneic transplant as initial postremission therapy. Moreover, different conditioning regimens have subsequently reduced the morbidity associated with BMT. According to the 2015 National Comprehensive Cancer Network guidelines, HDAC is appropriate consolidation for patients under age 60 with more favorable karyotypes/molecular findings and those who decline BMT, cannot undergo allogeneic BMT due to comorbidities, or lack a suitable donor.

Question

Is HDAC a reasonable treatment for patients with AML in CR?

Answer

Yes, although HDAC can be safely used as initial postremission therapy for consolidation, it is associated with higher relapse than BMT. Therefore, BMT should be strongly considered based on cytogenetic or molecular risk.

CHAPTER 54

GENOTYPE FOR RISK STRATIFICATION IN ACUTE MYELOID LEUKEMIA

Daniel O'Neil

Mutations and Treatment Outcome in Cytogenetically Normal Acute Myeloid Leukemia

Schlenk RF, Döhner K, Krauter J, et al. *N Engl J Med.* 2008;358(18):1909–1918

BACKGROUND

Despite its effectiveness in treating acute myeloid leukemia (AML) patients after initial remission, stem-cell transplantation (SCT) was generally reserved for those at highest risk of relapse due to significant treatment-related mortality. At the time of this study, several somatic gene mutations were suspected of having prognostic relevance in AML with a normal karyotype. Such mutations included those of the mixed-lineage leukemia (*MLL*), fms-related tyrosine kinase 3 (*FLT3*), nucleophosmin (*NPM1*), CCAAT/enhancer-binding protein α (*CEBPA*), and neuroblastoma RAS viral oncogene homolog (*NRAS*) genes.

OBJECTIVES

To assess the relationship of genetic mutations to treatment outcomes in normal-karyotype AML.

METHODS

Post hoc retrospective analysis of patients with normal-karyotype AML from 4 previously completed prospective treatment trials from 1993 to 2004.

Patients

872 patients. Inclusion criteria included AML with a normal karyotype.

Interventions

Blood or bone marrow specimens were screened for gene fusions and mutations (*FLT3*-ITD/TKD, *CEBPA*, *MLL*, *NPM1*, and *NRAS* genes, among others). Each trial protocol included the same induction and first cycle of postremission chemotherapy. Patients with an HLA-matched related donor subsequently underwent allogeneic SCT. Unmatched patients received further chemotherapy or were randomized to further chemotherapy or autologous SCT.

Outcomes

The primary outcome was relapse-free survival (RFS) at 4 years, defined as the lack of relapse or death among patients who achieved complete remission (CR). Secondary outcomes were CR after induction and overall survival (OS).

KEY RESULTS

- 668/872 patients (77%) achieved CR. Mutations in *NPM1* without *FLT3*-ITD and in *CEBPA* were associated with CR (OR 1.48, 95% CI 1.21–1.80 and OR 1.33, 95% CI 1.01–1.74, respectively).
- Among patients achieving CR, mutations in *CEBPA* as well as *NPM1* without *FLT3*-ITD were associated with greater RFS (HR 0.48, 95% CI 0.30–0.75 and HR 0.44, 95% CI 0.32–0.61, respectively) and OS (HR 0.50, 95% CI 0.30–0.83 and HR 0.51, 95% CI 0.37–0.70, respectively).
- Among patients with mutations in *NPM1* without *FLT3*-ITD, there was no statistically significant difference in RFS between those with and without a matched donor; improved OS was seen in patients with a matched donor in other genotypes, excluding mutations in *CEBPA* (HR 0.61, 95% CI 0.40–0.94).

STUDY CONCLUSIONS

New cases of AML with normal cytogenetics and mutations in *CEBPA* or in *NPM1* without *FLT3*-ITD should be considered favorable risk and may not benefit from SCT.

COMMENTARY

This study influenced postremission treatment recommendations for AML patients with a normal karyotype by demonstrating improved clinical outcomes in 2 specific genotypes: biallelic mutations to *CEBPA* and mutations of *NPM1* without *FLT3*-ITD. It was one of the first studies that correlated a wide array of genetic mutations and prognosis after treatment, ushering in an era in which treatment recommendations for AML are based on molecular markers. Caveats include the use of retrospective data for analysis and the use of data from 4 separate trials. However, subsequent prospective studies have confirmed these links to outcomes. Further research has begun to elucidate the role of many other mutations. The list of markers recommended for evaluation by the 2016 National Comprehensive Cancer Network guidelines for new AML patients continues to include *CEBPA*, *NPM1,* and *FLT3*-ITD, among many others.

Question

Should patients with normal-karyotype AML be offered genetic testing for risk stratification?

Answer

Yes, the presence of mutations in *NPM1* without *FLT3*-ITD and in *CEBPA* confers a more favorable prognosis, and is commonly used to inform decisions around risk-based chemotherapy or bone marrow transplant regimens.

INFECTIOUS DISEASES

CHAPTER 55	# ART FOR EARLY ASYMPTOMATIC HIV: THE START STUDY

Ersilia M. DeFilippis

Initiation of Antiretroviral Therapy in Early Asymptomatic HIV Infection

Lundgren JD, Babiker AG, Gordin F, et al. *N Engl J Med.* 2015;373(9):795–807

BACKGROUND

In contrast to strong evidence for antiretroviral therapy (ART) in patients with lower CD4 counts, at the time of this study recommendations for those with higher counts were of variable strength and often relied upon inconsistent observational data with limited follow-up. Given uncertainty about whether the benefits to asymptomatic patients with comparatively robust immune systems outweighed the costs and potential toxicity, a randomized trial of ART in early HIV was necessary.

OBJECTIVES

To determine the benefit and safety of initiating ART in asymptomatic HIV-positive patients with CD4 counts >500 cells/mm^3.

METHODS

Randomized controlled trial at 215 sites in 35 countries on 6 continents from 2009 to 2013.

Patients

4,685 healthy HIV-positive adult patients. Inclusion criteria included age ≥18 years, CD4 count >500 cells/mm^3. Exclusion criteria included any previous ART, history of AIDS, or current pregnancy or breastfeeding.

Intervention

Immediate initiation versus deferred initiation of ART. In the deferred initiation group, ART was started when CD4 count fell below 350 cells/mm^3 or upon development of a condition necessitating ART initiation (including AIDS-defining conditions or pregnancy). Median follow-up time was 2.8 years.

Outcomes

The primary outcome was a composite of both serious AIDS-related events (modified AIDS-defining conditions or AIDS mortality) and serious non–AIDS-related events (including cardiovascular disease, end-stage renal disease, hepatic disease, non–AIDS-defining malignancy, or non-AIDS mortality). Secondary outcomes included the individual components of the composite outcome, all-cause mortality, and unscheduled hospitalizations.

KEY RESULTS

- The composite primary outcome occurred in fewer patients in the immediate initiation group (42 vs. 96, HR 0.43, 95% CI 0.30–0.62, $p < 0.001$).
- Fewer patients in the immediate initiation group experienced serious AIDS-related events (14 vs. 50, HR = 0.28, 95% CI 0.15–0.50, $p < 0.001$) and serious non–AIDS-related events (29 vs. 47, HR = 0.61, 95% CI 0.38–0.97, $p = 0.04$).
- There were no statistically significant differences in death from any cause ($p = 0.13$) or unscheduled hospitalizations ($p = 0.28$).

STUDY CONCLUSIONS

Immediate initiation of ART is beneficial for patients with CD4 counts >500 cells/mm^3.

COMMENTARY

The START study, which was terminated early for efficacy in the immediate initiation group, was remarkable for both its large size and broad generalizability. Along with the TEMPRANO trial,[1] which was published at the same time, START definitively proved the value of early ART initiation for those with higher CD4 counts. Collectively, this evidence immediately influenced the 2016 US Department and Health and Human Services ART guidelines to strongly recommend ART for all.

Question

Should HIV-positive patients with a CD4 count >500 cells/mm^3 start ART?

Answer

Yes, early initiation of ART is associated with fewer serious AIDS- and non–AIDS-related events.

References

1. Danel C, Moh R, Gabillard D, et al; TEMPRANO ANRS 12136 Study Group. A Trial of Early Antiretrovirals and Isoniazid Preventive Therapy in Africa. *N Engl J Med.* 2015;373(9):808–822.

CHAPTER 56

DIRECT ACTING ANTIVIRALS FOR HCV: THE NEUTRINO AND FISSION TRIALS

Michelle Jose-Kampfner

Sofosbuvir for Previously Untreated Chronic Hepatitis C Infection

Lawitz E, Mangia A, Wyles D, et al. *N Engl J Med*. 2013;368(20):1878–1887

BACKGROUND

Prior to 2011, standard treatment for most patients with hepatitis C virus (HCV) was pegylated interferon and ribavirin for 9 to 12 months – a frequently ineffective treatment fraught with dose-limiting side effects. Direct-acting antivirals (DAAs) offered the promise of tolerable and effective therapy, but first-generation drugs, boceprevir and telaprevir, were limited by low-resistance thresholds, adverse reactions, limited genotypic spectra, and drug interactions. The second-generation DAA, sofosbuvir, offered a potentially more effective and safer treatment option.

OBJECTIVES

To evaluate efficacy and safety of sofosbuvir-based therapy in previously untreated HCV patients.

	NEUTRINO	FISSION
Methods	Single-group, open-label study at 56 sites across the United States in 2012	Randomized, open-label, active-control, noninferiority trial conducted in 97 sites across the United States, Australia, and Europe from 2011 to 2012
Patients	Inclusion criteria included age ≥18 years and HCV RNA ≥10^4 copies. Exclusion criteria included significant non-HCV liver disease and psychiatric comorbidity	
	327 patients, mostly HCV genotype 1 or 4, reflective of the general population. It comprised patients with historically lower treatment responses, including African Americans and those with cirrhosis and non-CC IL 28B genotypes	499 patients with genotypes 2 and 3, including a significant proportion of cirrhotic individuals
Intervention	Sofosbuvir (400 mg daily) plus peginterferon-ribavirin for 12 weeks versus adjusted historical control	12 weeks of sofosbuvir (400 mg daily) plus ribavirin or 24 weeks of peginterferon-ribavirin

	NEUTRINO	**FISSION**
Outcomes	The primary outcome was sustained virologic response (SVR, undetectable HCV viral load 12 weeks after the end of treatment). Secondary outcomes included side effects	
Key Results	More patients receiving sofosbuvir-peginterferon-ribavirin experienced SVR compared to the adjusted historical control (90% vs. 60%, $p < 0.001$)	67% of patients achieved SVR in both the sofosbuvir-ribavirin and peginterferon-ribavirin groups ($p < 0.001$ for noninferiority). Adverse events were less frequent in the sofosbuvir group (no p values reported), including flu-like symptoms (3% vs. 18%) and depression (5% vs. 14%)

STUDY CONCLUSIONS

NEUTRINO demonstrated the efficacy of adding sofosbuvir to the gold standard treatment. FISSION showed noninferiority of a shorter, interferon-free, sofosbuvir-based regimen with fewer side effects.

COMMENTARY

This landmark article was published alongside another study that demonstrated impressive SVRs with the addition of sofosbuvir for patients without other treatment options.[1] These initial trials paved the way for subsequent evaluations of new DAAs, leading to a revolution in HCV treatment from difficult and lengthy regimens to shorter, easily administered, well-tolerated therapies; while eradication of HCV was previously rare, DAAs have led to the potential to cure almost all patients. This dramatic change is reflected in the 2016 joint Infectious Diseases Society of America and American Association for the Study of Liver Disease HCV treatment guidelines, which recommend therapy for essentially all patients using sofosbuvir and other DAAs while minimizing ribavirin and interferon.

Question

Are DAA-based regimens an appropriate treatment choice for HCV?

Answer

Yes, later-generation DAAs are extremely effective and better tolerated than traditional interferon-based regimens.

References

1. Jacobson IM, Gordon SC, Kowdley KV, et al. Sofosbuvir for hepatitis C genotype 2 or 3 in patients without treatment options. *N Engl J Med.* 2013;368(20):1867–1877.

CHAPTER 57

ANTIBIOTIC MONOTHERAPY FOR FEBRILE NEUTROPENIA

Sarah E. Post

A Randomized Trial Comparing Ceftazidime Alone With Combination Antibiotic Therapy in Cancer Patients With Fever and Neutropenia

Pizzo PA, Hathorn JW, Hiemenz J, et al. *N Engl J Med*. 1986;315(9):552–558

BACKGROUND

Studies in the early 1980s showed that rapid initiation of broad-spectrum antibiotics improved outcomes in febrile neutropenia. Almost all these studies evaluated combinations of antibiotics, often with high toxicity. The introduction of broad-spectrum antipseudomonal cephalosporins raised the question of whether empiric treatment with a single agent could achieve similar results while reducing toxicity and cost.

OBJECTIVES

To compare the efficacy of single-agent antibiotic treatment against standard combination therapy for initial management of febrile neutropenia.

METHODS

Randomized controlled trial over 38 months at a single American cancer center.

Patients

318 adult and pediatric cancer patients experiencing a total of 550 episodes of febrile neutropenia. Neutropenia was defined as absolute neutrophil count $<500/mm^3$ or between 500 and 1,000 but expected to decline to $<500/mm^3$. Exclusion criteria were penicillin allergy or receipt of any antibiotics in the 72 hours preceding enrollment.

Interventions

Ceftazidime (90 mg/kg in 3 divided doses) versus combination therapy (cephalothin – a first-generation cephalosporin, gentamicin, and carbenicillin). The initial regimen was continued until 1 of 3 criteria was met: resolution of both fever and neutropenia, isolation of a pathogen, or a change in clinical status warranting regimen modification.

Outcomes

The primary outcomes were survival at 72 hours and until resolution of neutropenia. Results were stratified by presence of documented infection versus unexplained cause of fever. Secondary outcomes included microbiologic outcomes, toxicity, and the proportion of patients whose treatments were modified.

KEY RESULTS

- At 72 hours, 189/190 (99%) of patients with unexplained fevers in the ceftazidime group were alive versus 204/204 (100%) in the combination group; among those with documented infections, 98% survived to 72 hours in both groups (90/92 and 63/64, respectively).
- Survival to resolution of neutropenia was similar across groups. Survival was 98% in both the ceftazidime and combination groups (186/190 and 199/204, respectively) among patients with unexplained fevers and approximately 90% among those with documented infection (82/92 and 58/64, respectively).
- Hepatotoxicity was less frequent in the ceftazidime group (3% vs. 16%, $p < 0.001$).

STUDY CONCLUSIONS

Treatment with ceftazidime was as effective as a combination regimen for initial management of neutropenic fever among cancer patients.

COMMENTARY

This was the first large trial to compare single-agent to standard multiagent empiric treatment of cancer patients with neutropenic fever. Though the study was criticized for the frequency of regimen modification (most commonly the addition of another antibiotic), the practice arguably reflects the real-world experience of managing patients whose complex clinical courses require frequent reassessment. These results, along with those of later trials, led to a recommendation of single-agent antipseudomonal cephalosporin as a first-line empiric option in the 1997 Infectious Diseases Society of America neutropenic fever guidelines. In the current 2011 guidelines, all first-line options for high-risk patients are monotherapies, and ceftazidime remains one of the recommended initial choices.

Question

Is empiric treatment with a single broad-spectrum antibiotic a reasonable initial choice for neutropenic patients with fever?

Answer

Yes, empiric treatment with an antipseudomonal cephalosporin works as well as a combination regimen in febrile neutropenia, assuming appropriate modification of the regimen based on clinical course.

HIV PRE-EXPOSURE CHEMOPROPHYLAXIS: THE iPrEx STUDY

CHAPTER 58

Michelle Jose-Kampfner

Preexposure Chemoprophylaxis for HIV Prevention in Men Who Have Sex With Men
Grant RM, Lama JR, Anderson PL, et al; iPrEx Study Team. *N Engl J Med*. 2010;
363(27):2587–2599

BACKGROUND

At the time of this study, biomedical HIV prevention science lagged behind advances in treatment. While antiretroviral postexposure chemoprophylaxis had long been recommended for contact with HIV-positive fluids, and there were initial reports of efficacy for preventive vaginal microbicidal gel, it was unknown whether oral antiretrovirals could be used routinely for pre-exposure chemoprophylaxis (PrEP).

OBJECTIVES

To evaluate the efficacy and safety of daily PrEP in men who have sex with men (MSM), a group at high risk for HIV infection.

METHODS

Randomized, double-blind, controlled trial at 11 sites in North and South America, Asia, Australia, and Africa between 2007 and 2009.

Patients

2,499 MSM. Inclusion criteria included male sex at birth, age ≥18 years, HIV-negative status, high risk for HIV acquisition based on hazardous sexual activities during the preceding 6 months, and normal (or near-normal) serum chemistry and hematologic tests. Exclusion criteria included serious and active illness. Patient characteristics were well balanced except for age (mean age for the treatment group was 9 months older than that of the placebo group).

Interventions

FTC-TDF (daily combination pill of emtricitabine/tenofovir disoproxil fumarate) versus placebo. All patients underwent study visits every 4 weeks for drug dispensation, adherence monitoring and counseling, medical history, and HIV testing. Patients also received frequent screening for high-risk behaviors and sexually transmitted infections, as well as intermittent safety labs.

Outcomes

The primary outcome was HIV seroconversion. Secondary outcomes included adverse events (both severe and nonsevere). A prespecified case-control analysis was performed to assess the effect of drug levels on risk of seroconversion.

KEY RESULTS

- More patients in the placebo group experienced HIV seroconversion (64 vs. 36, RRR 44%, 95% CI 15%–63%, p = 0.005).
- There were no statistically significant differences in severe adverse effects (p = 0.57) or the need for drug discontinuation across groups (p = 0.82). The treatment group had a higher rate of nausea (22 events vs. 10 events, p = 0.04) and unintentional weight loss (34 events vs. 19 events, p = 0.04).
- Within the treatment group, drug levels were detectable in 9% of those who acquired HIV and 51% of those who remained HIV negative, and patients with detectable drug levels had a 92% RRR (95% CI 40%–99%, p < 0.001) for HIV acquisition compared to those with undetectable levels.

STUDY CONCLUSIONS

PrEP with daily FTC-TDF safely and effectively reduces the risk of HIV acquisition in MSM, particularly among those with good adherence.

COMMENTARY

iPrEx was a landmark study that demonstrated a safe and efficacious strategy to prevent HIV in a particularly vulnerable, high-risk group. Subsequent trials have shown benefit for PrEP in multiple other populations and settings, including a recent study that showed efficacy with intermittent, on-demand PrEP before and after high-risk intercourse. As a result, the Centers for Disease Control and Prevention now recommends daily PrEP for high-risk populations.[1]

Question

Is PrEP effective in preventing HIV seroconversion?

Answer

Yes, PrEP with daily FTC-TDF is well tolerated and prevents HIV in multiple high-risk populations.

References

1. US Public Health Service. Preexposure prophylaxis for the prevention of HIV infection in the United States - 2014: A clinical practice guideline. www.cdc.gov/hiv/pdf/prepguidelines2014.pdf. Accessed April 7, 2016.

CHAPTER 59

ORAL VANCOMYCIN FOR SEVERE *C. DIFFICILE* INFECTIONS

Sarah E. Post

A Comparison of Vancomycin and Metronidazole for the Treatment of Clostridium difficile-Associated Diarrhea, Stratified by Disease Severity

Zar FA, Bakkanagari SR, Moorthi KM, Davis MB. *Clin Infect Dis*. 2007;45(3):302–307

BACKGROUND

At the time of this study, metronidazole and vancomycin were the most common antibiotic treatments for *Clostridium difficile*-associated diarrhea (CDAD). Two prospective randomized trials had compared the drugs, and while they found no difference in efficacy, both were small and neither was blinded or placebo controlled. No prior study had stratified patients by disease severity.

OBJECTIVES

To evaluate whether metronidazole or vancomycin was more effective in treating mild or severe CDAD.

METHODS

Prospective, randomized, double-blind, double-dummy, placebo-controlled trial conducted at a single American hospital between 1994 and 2002. Randomization was stratified by disease severity.

Patients

150 patients. Inclusion criteria included diarrhea and either positive *C. difficile* toxin A or pseudomembranous colitis on endoscopy. Exclusion criteria included recent administration of either study drug, prior failure of either study drug, or very severe complications such as bowel perforation or obstruction. Patients who had pseudomembranous colitis, required ICU treatment, or met ≥2 predetermined criteria (age, fever, low albumin, or white blood cell count >15,000/dL) were considered to have "severe" infection.

Interventions

Metronidazole tablets (250 mg 4 times daily) plus placebo liquid versus oral vancomycin liquid (125 mg 4 times daily) plus placebo tablets.

Outcomes

The 3 coprimary outcomes were *C. difficile* cure rate (resolution of diarrhea by day 6 of treatment and negative toxin at days 6 and 10), treatment failure (persistence of diarrhea for 6 days or more, toxin positivity at day 6, need for colectomy, or death any time after 5 days of treatment), and relapse (recurrence of toxin-positive diarrhea by day 21 after initial cure).

KEY RESULTS

- The overall cure rate was 84% (66/79) in the metronidazole group and 97% (69/71) in the vancomycin group ($p = 0.006$).
- Among the 81 patients with mild disease, the cure rates for metronidazole and vancomycin were not statistically significantly different (90% vs. 98%, $p = 0.36$).
- Among the 69 patients with severe disease, the cure rate was lower with metronidazole (76% vs. 97%, $p = 0.02$).
- There was no statistically significant difference in the rate of relapse ($p = 0.27$).

STUDY CONCLUSIONS

Vancomycin was superior to metronidazole overall for treating CDAD, with the benefit limited to patients with severe disease.

COMMENTARY

This was the first blinded, placebo-controlled trial to demonstrate that oral vancomycin is superior for some patients with CDAD. It was criticized for outcomes based on microbiologic cure rather than just symptomatic resolution as relied upon in clinical practice. However, toxin positivity alone was a cause of treatment failure for only 2 patients and thus unlikely to have significantly influenced the findings. Subsequent studies have confirmed the superiority of vancomycin for severe infection. The 2010 Infectious Diseases Society of America *Clostridium difficile* guidelines recommend risk stratification for all patients and vancomycin as first-line treatment for severe CDAD.

Question

Is there a preferred antimicrobial agent for treating severe CDAD?

Answer

Yes, vancomycin is more effective than metronidazole in these cases.

CHAPTER 60

SMX-TMP FOR PCP PROPHYLAXIS IN AIDS

Michelle Jose-Kampfner ■ Sarah E. Post

Safety and Efficacy of Sulfamethoxazole and Trimethoprim Chemoprophylaxis for Pneumocystis carinii Pneumonia in AIDS

Fischl MA, Dickinson GM, La Voie L. *JAMA*. 1988;259(8):1185–1189

BACKGROUND

In the 1980s, Kaposi sarcoma (KS) and *Pneumocystis carinii* pneumonia (PCP, now known as *Pneumocystis jiroveci*) were defining features of the acquired immune deficiency syndrome (AIDS). Over 50% of AIDS patients developed PCP, which was associated with high mortality. Sulfamethoxazole and trimethoprim (SMX-TMP) had been used to treat PCP in AIDS and other immunocompromised patients and (at a lower dose) to prevent PCP recurrence, but had not been studied as a measure to prevent first PCP occurrence.

OBJECTIVES

To determine the safety, tolerability, and efficacy of SMX-TMP to prevent PCP in patients with AIDS.

METHODS

Randomized controlled trial conducted between 1984 and 1987.

Patients

60 patients. The inclusion criterion was AIDS with newly diagnosed KS. Exclusion criteria included previous or active opportunistic infections, prior antiretroviral therapy, and prior PCP chemoprophylaxis.

Interventions

SMX-TMP (800/160 mg twice daily) with leucovorin versus control group. Patients were followed for at least 24 months.

Outcomes

The primary outcome was the development of PCP. Secondary outcomes included survival and adverse effects.

KEY RESULTS

- No patients developed PCP while receiving prophylaxis, though 4 of 5 who stopped SMX-TMP due to toxicity later developed the infection. PCP occurred in 53% of the control group.
- The SMX-TMP group had longer median survival (20 months vs. 11 months).

- 81% of patients who developed PCP had CD4 counts ≤200 cells/mm^3 at study entry.
- 50% of patients in the SMX-TMP group experienced an adverse reaction (most commonly rash) and 17% discontinued the regimen due to an adverse reaction.

STUDY CONCLUSIONS

SMX-TMP prevents PCP infection in patients with AIDS-associated KS, increases length of survival, and is generally tolerable.

COMMENTARY

At the time of this study, AIDS was a poorly understood illness that resulted in rapid and inevitable mortality, often from PCP. Despite its small size, unclear generalizability to other AIDS populations, and concern that the development of drug intolerance and microbial resistance would make treating PCP infections more difficult, this trial demonstrated a dramatic benefit and resulted in important practice changes. In 1989, the Centers for Disease Control released its first HIV-related treatment guideline and recommended PCP prophylaxis for those with CD4 counts <200 cells/mm^3, a recommendation that has since been expanded to include multiple features of advanced HIV (e.g., certain AIDS-defining illnesses) in the 2016 Infectious Diseases Society of America opportunistic infection guidelines.

Question

Should patients with advanced HIV receive SMX-TMP prophylaxis?

Answer

Yes, SMX-TMP prophylaxis prevents PCP and improves survival.

CHAPTER 61

COMBINATION ART FOR HIV

Sarah E. Post

A Trial Comparing Nucleoside Monotherapy With Combination Therapy in HIV-Infected Adults With CD4 Cell Counts From 200 to 500 per Cubic Millimeter.

Hammer SM, Katzenstein DA, Hughes MD, et al. *N Engl J Med*. 1996;335(15): 1081–1090

BACKGROUND

The first antiretroviral treatment for HIV, zidovudine (also known as AZT) monotherapy, had been shown to improve survival and slow disease progression, but its effects waned rapidly with prolonged treatment. At the time of this study, combinations of zidovudine and newly developed nucleoside reverse transcriptase inhibitors, zalcitabine and didanosine, had shown improvement in laboratory markers of disease, though their impact on clinical outcomes was unclear.

OBJECTIVES

To compare treatment effectiveness of nucleoside monotherapy versus nucleoside combination therapy.

METHODS

Randomized, double-blind, placebo-controlled trial at 52 sites in the United States and Puerto Rico between 1991 and 1992.

Patients

2,467 patients with HIV-1 infection, 43% of whom had never received antiretroviral therapy. Inclusion criteria included CD4 count between 200 and 500 per mm^3 and age ≥12 years. Exclusion criteria included history of AIDS-defining illness other than minimal mucocutaneous Kaposi sarcoma.

Interventions

There were 4 treatment groups: zidovudine alone versus zidovudine and zalcitabine versus zidovudine and didanosine versus didanosine alone. Patients were followed for a median of 143 weeks.

Outcomes

The primary outcome was a composite of >50% decline in pretreatment CD4 count, AIDS-defining illness, or death. Secondary outcomes included death or a composite of AIDS or death.

KEY RESULTS

- In the zidovudine alone group, 32% of patients reached the primary outcome versus 18% in the zidovudine plus didanosine group, 20% in the zidovudine plus zalcitabine group, and 22% in the didanosine alone group ($p < 0.001$ for each paired comparison to zidovudine alone).
- 16% of patients in the zidovudine alone group died or developed AIDS versus 11% ($p = 0.005$), 12% ($p = 0.085$), and 11% ($p = 0.019$) in the zidovudine plus didanosine, zidovudine plus zalcitabine, and didanosine alone groups, respectively. 9% of patients in the zidovudine group died, versus 5% ($p = 0.008$), 7% ($p = 0.10$), and 5% ($p = 0.003$), respectively.
- 53% of patients prematurely discontinued treatment, only 7% of whom stopped due to adverse events that required discontinuation by study protocol.

STUDY CONCLUSIONS

Treatment with zidovudine plus didanosine, zidovudine plus zalcitabine, or didanosine alone was superior to zidovudine alone at slowing HIV disease progression among patients with CD4 counts between 200 and 500.

COMMENTARY

This trial was the first to establish the superiority of combination ART to improve HIV outcomes, setting the conceptual course for future advances. Along with a subgroup analysis of this trial, it also demonstrated the modest correlation between clinical outcomes and surrogate endpoints (e.g., CD4 count, viral load) that have become accepted clinical trial outcomes and the focus of monitoring in clinical practice. The rapid, subsequent development of additional antiretroviral drugs and classes led to numerous novel multidrug regimens that are now in use. Nonetheless, along with the contemporaneous Delta study[1] – which showed similar results in patients with more advanced disease – this trial remains notable for confirming the promise of new antiretrovirals and combination therapy.

Question

Should patients with HIV receive zidovudine monotherapy?

Answer

No, 2-drug regimens result in better outcomes than monotherapy, although multiple-drug regimens are now standard of care.

References

1. Delta Coordinating Committee. Delta: A randomised double-blind controlled trial comparing combinations of zidovudine plus didanosine or zalcitabine with zidovudine alone in HIV-infected individuals. *Lancet.* 1996;348(9023):283–291.

CHAPTER 62

EARLY ART TO PREVENT HIV TRANSMISSION

Sarah E. Post

Prevention of HIV-1 Infection With Early Antiretroviral Therapy

Cohen MS, Chen YQ, McCauley M, et al. *N Engl J Med*. 2011;365(6):493–505

BACKGROUND

By the time of this study, antiretroviral therapy (ART) had been definitively shown to improve survival among patients with advanced HIV. Because ART frequently led to significant viral suppression, it was theorized that treatment could reduce transmission to seronegative individuals. This effect had been demonstrated in observational studies but not in randomized trials.

OBJECTIVES

To assess whether ART could reduce HIV transmission in serodiscordant couples and to evaluate its effect on clinical outcomes in infected persons with moderate CD4 counts.

METHODS

Randomized controlled trial at 13 sites in Africa, Asia, and the United States between 2007 and 2010.

Patients

1,763 serodiscordant couples who were required to be in stable, sexually active relationships (≥3 months in duration and expected to be maintained). The HIV-infected partner was required to have a baseline CD4 count between 350 and 550 cells/mm^3, no prior ART use (with exception of short-term prevention of mother-to-child transmission), and no history of AIDS-defining illness. Exclusion criteria included injection drug use within 5 years.

Interventions

Early ART (HIV-infected partners starting treatment at enrollment) versus delayed ART (HIV-infected partners starting treatment when CD4 count fell below 250 or at occurrence of an AIDS-related illness).

Outcomes

The primary prevention outcome was genotypically linked HIV transmission to HIV-negative partners. A secondary outcome was any new HIV infection in HIV-negative partners. The primary clinical outcome was the earliest occurrence in the HIV-infected participants of pulmonary TB, severe bacterial infection, any World Health Organization stage 4 event, or death.

KEY RESULTS

- 28 linked HIV transmissions occurred: 1 in the early ART group and 27 in the late ART group (HR 0.04, 95% CI 0.01–0.27, p < 0.001). Each linked transmission in the delayed ART group occurred while the HIV-infected participant was not receiving ART.
- Early ART reduced the rate of all HIV transmission: 4 seroconversions occurred in the early group versus 35 in the delayed group (HR 0.11, 95% CI 0.04–0.32, p < 0.001).
- The primary clinical outcome occurred in 40 individuals in the early group versus 65 in the delayed group (HR 0.59, 95% CI 0.40–0.88, p = 0.01).

STUDY CONCLUSIONS

Early ART for HIV-positive partners with CD4 counts between 350 and 550 cells/ mm^3 reduced HIV transmission in serodiscordant couples and reduced morbidity for the HIV-infected participants.

COMMENTARY

This trial demonstrated that ART could dramatically reduce HIV transmission, possibly more effectively than most existing prevention strategies. The outcomes among the HIV-infected partners also added randomized, prospective data to support the controversial hypothesis that earlier provision of ART could prevent serious illness in this population. Together, these findings imply that widespread ART provision holds promise as a strategy to contain or even end the epidemic. Caveats include limited enrollment of men who have sex with men and exclusion of injection drug users. The trial's remarkable findings led to important practice changes and an update to the 2016 US Health and Human Services antiretroviral therapy guidelines, which now recommend initiation of ART for all HIV-infected patients specifically to prevent sexual transmission.

Question

Does early ART provision prevent HIV transmission to a seronegative partner?

Answer

Yes, ART substantially reduces the rate of HIV transmission within serodiscordant couples.

CHAPTER 63

TIMING OF ART WITH ACUTE OIs IN HIV

Sarah E. Post

Early Antiretroviral Therapy Reduces AIDS Progression/Death in Individuals With Acute Opportunistic Infections: A Multicenter Randomized Strategy Trial

Zolopa AR, Andersen J, Komarow L, et al. *PLoS ONE*. 2009;4(5):e5575

BACKGROUND

Many HIV patients first present to medical care upon developing serious bacterial infections (SBIs) or AIDS-defining opportunistic infections (OIs). At the time of this study, optimal timing for starting antiretroviral therapy (ART) in these patients was uncertain, and concern remained that starting ART while treating the presenting condition could result in increased drug toxicity or drug–drug interactions, reduce ART adherence due to polypharmacy, or increase the frequency and morbidity of immune reconstitution inflammatory syndrome (IRIS).

OBJECTIVES

To evaluate whether early ART was associated with improved outcomes compared to deferred ART among patients presenting with SBIs or AIDS-related OIs.

METHODS

Randomized, open-label controlled trial at 39 US sites and 1 site in South Africa between 2003 and 2006.

Patients

282 patients. Inclusion criteria included HIV infection, age >13 years, and either an SBI with CD4 count <200 cells/mm^3 or an AIDS-defining OI. Treatment for the qualifying SBI or OI had to have begun within 14 days of randomization. Exclusion criteria included tuberculosis or a history of recent or significant ART exposure.

Interventions

Early ART (expected to start ART within 48 hours of study enrollment) versus deferred ART (encouraged to start between 6 and 12 weeks after enrollment). Regimen choice and exact timing were left to individual clinicians.

Outcomes

The primary outcome was a 3-level ordered categorical variable at week 48: no progression with complete viral suppression (best), no progression with incomplete viral suppression (intermediate), and AIDS progression or death (worst). Secondary outcomes included adverse events, including IRIS, and a composite of AIDS progression or death.

KEY RESULTS

- The rates of the primary outcome were similar between early and deferred ART groups (best 47.5% vs. 44.7%, intermediate 38.3% vs. 31.2%, worst 14.2% vs. 24.1%, $p = 0.22$).
- The early ART group had a lower risk for AIDS progression or death (HR 0.53, 95% CI = 0.30–0.92, $p = 0.02$).
- There was a higher rate of neutropenia in the deferred ART group ($p = 0.05$), but no statistically significant differences in other adverse events.

STUDY CONCLUSIONS

Early initiation of ART among HIV-positive patients presenting with SBI or OIs reduced AIDS progression and mortality and did not result in more adverse events than a deferred ART strategy.

COMMENTARY

This was the first large trial to assess the safety of starting ART in patients presenting with a broad variety of SBIs or AIDS-defining OIs. Although it failed to show a significant difference in the primary outcome, the study demonstrated clear benefit for early treatment in preventing AIDS progression or death, primarily by reducing the frequency of these outcomes soon after initiation. Caveats include enrollment of patients mainly in the United States rather than resource-limited settings, exclusion of tuberculosis patients, and relatively low prevalence of cryptococcus. Other trials have since shown mixed results for a few particular infections, such as tuberculous meningitis (equivocal) and cryptococcal meningitis (harm), where deferred ART is the strategy of choice. As a result of these studies, early ART is now standard of care for patients presenting with OIs other than cryptococcal and tuberculous meningitis, as reflected in the 2016 US Department of Health and Human Services ART treatment guidelines.

Question

Should patients who present with most SBIs and AIDS-related OIs be started on early ART?

Answer

Yes, with rare exceptions, ART started at the same time as treatment for these presenting conditions reduces AIDS progression or death compared with waiting until treatment completion.

CHAPTER 64

OSELTAMIVIR FOR INFLUENZA

Michelle Jose-Kampfner ■ Sarah E. Post

Use of the Oral Neuraminidase Inhibitor Oseltamivir in Experimental Human Influenza: Randomized Controlled Trials for Prevention and Treatment

Hayden FG, Treanor JJ, Fritz RS, et al. *JAMA*. 1999;282(13):1240–1246

BACKGROUND

At the time of this study, there were few effective medications for preventing the spread of influenza or treating established infection. Neuraminidase inhibitors showed promise for treatment, though the first drug in the class, zanamivir, was impractical given its intranasal route of delivery, which can worsen respiratory bronchospasm. The efficacy of the oral neuraminidase inhibitor, oseltamivir, was unknown.

OBJECTIVES

To measure safety, tolerability, and efficacy of oseltamivir for preventing and treating influenza.

METHODS

Two randomized, double-blind, placebo-controlled, dose-ranging trials – 1 prophylaxis, 1 treatment – conducted at 2 US centers in 1997.

Patients

102 healthy volunteers (33 in the prophylaxis study, 69 in the treatment study). Inclusion criteria included age 18 to 40 years and negative influenza antibody titers. Exclusion criteria included concurrent medication use or recent illness.

Interventions

Patients were isolated prior to, and 8 days after, being inoculated intranasally with influenza A. Prophylaxis study patients were randomized to receive various doses of oseltamivir or placebo starting 26 hours prior to inoculation and continuing for 5 days. Treatment study patients were randomized to receive various doses of oseltamivir or placebo beginning 28 hours after inoculation for 5 days.

Outcomes

Prophylaxis Study

The primary outcomes were frequency of viral infection (defined by a positive culture or increase in serum antibody titer) and viral shedding. Secondary outcomes included symptom scores and frequency of upper respiratory illness (URI).

Treatment Study

The primary outcome was quantity of virus shed over time in nasal washings. Secondary outcomes included time to cessation of shedding, symptom score, and time to alleviation of symptoms.

KEY RESULTS

- In the prophylaxis trial, 50% of placebo patients had viral shedding versus none in the pooled oseltamivir group ($p < 0.001$) and 67% of placebo patients had infection versus 38% in the treatment group ($p = 0.16$). 33% of placebo patients developed URI versus none in the oseltamivir group ($p = 0.01$).
- In the treatment trial, the combined oseltamivir group had less total viral shedding compared to the placebo group ($p = 0.02$), lower total symptom score ($p = 0.05$), and faster resolution of symptoms (53 hours vs. 95 hours, $p = 0.03$).

STUDY CONCLUSIONS

Prophylactic treatment with oral oseltamivir protected against viral shedding and symptoms of influenza. Treatment of infected subjects reduced viral shedding as well as severity and duration of illness.

COMMENTARY

Though it did not affect confirmed infection, this study was among the first to demonstrate that neuraminidase inhibitors could both prevent viral shedding and improve laboratory and clinical markers when used for treatment without observed dose-limiting intolerance. Subsequent trials demonstrating efficacy in naturally acquired influenza resulted in Food and Drug Administration approval for both prophylaxis (after exposure and during institutional outbreaks) and treatment, and oseltamivir remains widely used for these indications. The reduction of symptom duration with oseltamivir is modest, and there is controversy about its ability to prevent complications and hospitalizations. Nonetheless, due in part to this study's findings, the Infectious Diseases Society of America reinforced its recommendations to use neuraminidase inhibitors for prophylaxis and treatment in many high-risk groups and situations.

Question

Is it reasonable to provide influenza prophylaxis or treatment to high-risk patients?

Answer

Yes, oseltamivir prophylaxis prevents acquisition of influenza virus, and oseltamivir treatment reduces symptom burden and duration.

CHAPTER 65

INTENSITY OF RENAL REPLACEMENT THERAPY IN THE ICU

Mounica Vallurupalli

Intensity of Renal Support in Critically Ill Patients With Acute Kidney Injury

Palevsky PM, Zhang GH, O'Connor TK, et al. *N Engl J Med.* 2008;359(1):7–20

BACKGROUND

Critically ill patients with acute kidney injury (AKI) requiring renal replacement therapy (RRT) have mortality rates of approximately 50% to 70%. Prior to this trial, single-center studies reported inconsistent results about the relationship between mortality and intensity of RRT in the critically ill. Studies evaluating hemodialysis (HD) intensity often tested approaches that did not reflect clinical practice, with participants receiving only either HD or continuous venovenous hemofiltration (CVVH). No randomized data evaluating both options existed to guide clinical practice.

OBJECTIVES

To examine the effect of dialysis intensity on survival and recovery of kidney function in patients with critical illness and AKI.

METHODS

Randomized, parallel-group study at 27 US hospitals between 2003 and 2007.

Patients

1,124 patients. Inclusion criteria included age >18 years, AKI due to acute tubular necrosis, need for RRT, and sepsis or failure of 1 other organ. Exclusion criteria included chronic kidney disease, prior kidney transplant, and anticipated survival <28 days.

Interventions

Intensive therapy (HD 6 days/week or CVVH at 35 mL/kg/hr) versus usual intensity therapy (HD 3 days/week or CVVH at 20 mL/kg/hr). Within groups, decisions to initiate HD versus CVVH were determined using the Sepsis-related Organ Failure Assessment cardiovascular score. Patients were permitted to switch from HD to CVVH if hemodynamically unstable.

Outcomes

The primary outcome was all-cause mortality by day 60. Secondary outcomes included in-hospital death, recovery of kidney function (defined as a lack of need for continued dialysis with creatinine clearance ≥20 mL/min), duration of RRT, length of ICU and hospital stays, and days free from nonrenal organ failure. Complications included hypotension requiring vasopressor support.

KEY RESULTS
- 60-day all-cause mortality was similar in both groups (53.6% in the intensive therapy group vs. 51.5% in the low-intensity therapy group, $p = 0.47$).
- There were no statistically significant differences between the groups with respect to in-hospital death, recovery of kidney function, hospital- and ICU-free days, and organ-failure–free days.
- More patients in the intensive therapy group experienced hypotension requiring vasopressor support (14.4% vs. 10.0%, $p = 0.02$).

STUDY CONCLUSIONS
Intensive RRT in critically ill patients with AKI due to acute tubular necrosis does not decrease mortality when compared to usual intensity treatment.

COMMENTARY

This trial contrasted earlier studies that suggested a mortality benefit for high-intensity HD in patients with AKI requiring RRT. Caveats include enrollment of only patients with AKI due to ATN. The study's careful design ensured that the intensive therapy and usual intensity groups received different RRT regimens, and its findings helped resolve the debate regarding the utility of high-intensity RRT in critically ill patients. Subsequently, the RENAL study[1] evaluated high- and low-intensity CVVH and also demonstrated no difference in mortality or renal recovery. As a result of these 2 studies, the 2015 Kidney Disease Outcomes Quality Initiative dialysis guidelines do not endorse high-intensity RRT in any patient subgroup.

Question
Should patients with AKI and organ failure receive high-intensity RRT?

Answer
No, there is no evidence of benefit associated with this practice.

References
1. Bellomo R, Cass A, Cole L, et al; RENAL Replacement Therapy Study Investigators. Intensity of continuous renal replacement therapy in critically ill patients. *N Engl J Med.* 2009;361(17):1627–1638.

CHAPTER 66

ACE INHIBITORS IN CHRONIC NONDIABETIC NEPHROPATHY: THE REIN TRIAL

Julia Rudolf

Randomized Placebo-Controlled Trial of Effect of Ramipril on Decline in Glomerular Filtration Rate and Risk of Terminal Renal Failure in Proteinuric, Non-Diabetic Nephropathy

The GISEN Group. *Lancet.* 1997;349(9069):1857–1863

BACKGROUND

Prior to this study, angiotensin-converting enzyme (ACE) inhibitors were shown to be renoprotective among patients with diabetic nephropathy, demonstrating favorable effects on proteinuria and glomerular filtration rate (GFR) decline beyond those expected from blood pressure control alone. Given inconclusive results from existing studies, however, it remained unclear whether such benefits applied to nondiabetic nephropathies.

OBJECTIVES

To evaluate whether ACE inhibitors are superior to conventional blood pressure treatment for reducing proteinuria and progression of renal disease among patients with nondiabetic, proteinuric nephropathies.

METHODS

Randomized, double-blind, placebo-controlled trial with stratified randomization (based on baseline proteinuria) at 14 Italian hospitals. This analysis evaluated 1 of 2 patient strata (those with severe baseline proteinuria).

Patients

166 patients with normal or elevated blood pressure and baseline proteinuria >3 g/24 hr. Overall trial inclusion criteria included age 18 to 70 years, chronic nephropathy with persistent proteinuria (urinary protein excretion >1 g/24 hr for ≥3 months), and no ACE inhibition therapy for ≥2 months. Exclusion criteria included insulin-dependent diabetes, myocardial infarction or stroke within 6 months, severe uncontrolled hypertension (SBP ≥220 mm Hg and/or DBP ≥115 mm Hg), certain medications (e.g., nonsteroidal anti-inflammatory drugs), and evidence or suspicion of renovascular disease.

Interventions

Ramipril versus placebo. All patients also received other antihypertensive agents and recommendations to limit sodium intake, with treatment goal of DBP <90 mm Hg.

Outcomes

The primary outcome was rate of GFR decline. Secondary outcomes included degree of proteinuria, time to doubling of baseline serum creatinine or progression to end-stage renal failure (ESRF), and frequency of major cardiovascular (CV) complications.

KEY RESULTS

- Among 117 patients with ≥3 GFR evaluations, ramipril was associated with lower monthly GFR decline (0.53 mL/min vs. 0.88 mL/min, $p = 0.03$).
- Fewer patients in the ramipril group had doubling of serum creatinine or progression to ESRF (18 vs. 40, $p = 0.04$).
- Achieved mean systolic (144 mm Hg vs. 144.6 mm Hg, $p = 0.95$) and diastolic (88.2 mm Hg vs. 88.9 mm Hg, $p = 0.57$) blood pressure were similar.
- The number of nonfatal CV events requiring withdrawal from treatment was similar between the 2 groups.

STUDY CONCLUSIONS

In nondiabetic nephropathies with proteinuria of >3 g/24 hr, ramipril safely reduced proteinuria and GFR decline to an extent beyond that expected from blood pressure lowering alone.

COMMENTARY

REIN was pivotal for demonstrating the renoprotective effects of ACE inhibitors in nondiabetic patients with chronic nephropathy. The analysis of this stratum was terminated and reported early per protocol due to the significant benefit noted in the ramipril group. Caveats include the high proportion of men (85%) and small sample size. Evaluation of patients in the other stratum (those with baseline urine protein <3 g/24 hr) confirmed that ACE inhibitors also protect against progression to overt proteinuria and ESRF among those with less severe proteinuria.[1] Subsequent work advanced the REIN findings, showing that the benefits of ACE inhibitors are independent of initial GFR and particularly pronounced when initiated early among those with prominent proteinuria. Collectively, these findings led to the 2012 Kidney Disease Improving Global Outcomes blood pressure guidelines that recommend ACE inhibitors in proteinuric chronic kidney disease.

Question

Should ACE inhibitors be considered in patients with proteinuric chronic kidney disease?

Answer

Yes, ACE inhibitors possess renoprotective effects for patients with varying degrees of proteinuria.

References

1. Ruggenenti P, Perna A, Gherardi G, et al. Renoprotective properties of ACE-inhibition in non-diabetic nephropathies with non-nephrotic proteinuria. *Lancet.* 1999;354(9176):359–364.

CHAPTER 67

THE MDRD EQUATION TO ESTIMATE GFR

Julia Rudolf

A More Accurate Method to Estimate Glomerular Filtration Rate from Serum Creatinine: A New Prediction Equation.
Levey AS, Bosch JP, Lewis JB, et al. *Ann Intern Med.* 1999;130(6):461–470

BACKGROUND

Glomerular filtration rate (GFR) is considered the best index of renal function. However, direct measurement of GFR via urinary inulin clearance is cumbersome, and estimation by 24-hour urinary creatinine clearance overestimates GFR. Therefore, it is useful to estimate GFR using derived equations based on serum creatinine and other factors. Prior to this study, the Cockcroft–Gault equation was widely used despite the fact that it was derived from a small sample of male patients and included height and weight, variables which were often unavailable to laboratories.

OBJECTIVES

To develop an equation based on data from the Modification of Diet in Renal Disease (MDRD) study that would improve prediction of GFR from serum creatinine concentration and other factors.

METHODS

Cross-sectional retrospective analysis of data collected from patients with chronic kidney disease (CKD) who were enrolled in the MDRD study (a randomized controlled trial conducted in 15 clinical centers that evaluated the effect of protein restriction and blood pressure control on renal disease).

Patients

1,628 patients. 1,070 patients comprised the training sample and 558 comprised the validation sample.

Interventions

Seven equations were compared in the validation sample. The equations included Cockcroft–Gault, measured creatinine clearance, and 2 newly derived equations based on multivariate regression models (1 using demographic information as well as urine and serum biochemical values as covariates, and another using demographic information and serum biochemical values as covariates).

Outcomes

The primary outcome was the overall R^2 (a measure of model fit defined as the percentage of variability in log GFR explained) for each model. R^2 was calculated by comparing predicted and actual GFR values (measured via radioactive iothalamate clearance) in the validation sample.

KEY RESULTS

- The equation using demographic information and urine and serum biochemical values was associated with the maximal R^2 (91.2%), followed by the equation using demographic information and serum biochemical values (R^2 = 90.3%).
- The Cockcroft–Gault equation (R^2 = 84.2%) and creatinine clearance (R^2 = 86.6%) were less precise in predicting GFR.
- Higher serum creatinine, older age, female sex, nonblack ethnicity, higher BUN, and lower serum albumin were independently associated with lower GFR ($p < 0.001$ for all).

STUDY CONCLUSIONS

Both derived equations more accurately predict GFR than the Cockcroft–Gault equation or measured creatinine clearance.

COMMENTARY

In addition to their predictive ability, the 2 derived equations were the first to account for the effect of ethnicity, along with gender, age, and serum creatinine, on GFR – a feature not incorporated into other models up to that point. Although the equation that used urine values was more predictive of GFR, it was practically more difficult to use, and the model that does not use urine values is the one now referred to as the MDRD equation. Along with the CKD-EPI equation,[1] which was later validated in a larger, more diverse population of CKD patients and shown to be more accurate than the MDRD equation in the subset of patients with GFR >60 mL/min/m^2, the MDRD equation is currently used by most US chemistry laboratories.

Question

Is the MDRD equation an appropriate measure for estimating GFR in CKD patients?

Answer

Yes, although the CKD-EPI equation may be more accurate when the actual GFR is >60 mL/min/m^2.

References

1. Levey AS, Stevens LA, Schmid CH, et al; CKD-EPI (Cronic Kidney Disease Epidemiology Collaboration). A New Equation to Estimate Glomerular Filtration Rate. *Ann Intern Med.* 2009;150(9):604–612.

CHAPTER 68

HIGH-DOSE AND HIGH-FLUX MEMBRANE USE IN HEMODIALYSIS: THE HEMO STUDY

Julia Rudolf

Effect of Dialysis Dose and Membrane Flux in Maintenance Hemodialysis

Eknoyan G, Beck GJ, Cheung AK, et al. *N Engl J Med.* 2002;347(25):2010–2019

BACKGROUND

At the time of this study, the 5-year mortality rate of hemodialysis (HD) patients was 70%. The effects of high-dose HD (expressed as the equilibrated intradialytic urea reduction ratio, Kt/V) and high-flux membranes (membrane porosity estimated by degree of beta2-microglobulin clearance) on clinical outcomes in end-stage renal disease patients undergoing HD 3 times weekly were unclear. Small retrospective studies had produced conflicting results.

OBJECTIVES

To determine whether increasing dialysis dose or using high-flux membranes alters survival or morbidity in patients undergoing HD.

METHODS

Randomized trial with 2-by-2 factorial design at 15 US facilities associated with 72 dialysis centers between 1995 and 2000.

Patients

1,846 patients. Inclusion criteria included age 18 to 80 years and treatment with HD 3 times weekly for >3 months. Exclusion criteria included serum albumin <2.6 g/dL, inability to tolerate high-dose HD, and weight >100 kg.

Interventions

There were 2 comparisons: standard-dose (Kt/V of 1.05) versus high-dose (Kt/V of 1.45) dialysis and low-flux (beta2-microglobulin clearance <10 mL/min) versus high-flux (beta2-microglobulin clearance >20 mL/min) dialyzer.

Outcomes

The primary outcome was all-cause mortality. Main secondary outcomes included rate of all hospitalizations not related to vascular access and 3 composite outcomes: first hospitalization or death from any cause, first hospitalization for infection or death from any cause, and first decline of >15% from baseline serum albumin or death from any cause.

KEY RESULTS

- There were no statistically significant differences in the risk of all-cause mortality based on dialysis dose (RR 0.96, 95% CI 0.84–1.10, $p = 0.53$) or membrane flux (RR 0.92, 95% CI 0.81–1.05, $p = 0.23$).
- There were no statistically significant differences in the 4 main secondary outcomes based on dialysis dose or membrane flux.

STUDY CONCLUSIONS

High-dose HD or use of a high-flux membrane did not demonstrate benefit in patients undergoing HD 3 times weekly.

COMMENTARY

HEMO is considered the most comprehensive trial to date evaluating the effect of dose and flux (critical and potentially modifiable features of HD) in a population at very high risk for mortality. Caveats include difficulty recruiting patients and unaccounted effects of evolving HD technology on outcomes. While its primary and main secondary outcomes were negative, analyses suggesting subgroup effects (e.g., a 20% decrease of death from cardiac causes with the use of a high-flux membrane) led to further investigation targeting preselected groups. Subsequent trials showed a survival benefit with high-flux membranes in patients with low albumin (<4 g/dL) and in diabetic patients, while other studies confirmed a reduction in cardiovascular event-free survival. In turn, the 2015 Kidney Disease Outcomes Quality Initiative HD clinical practice guidelines report that there is insufficient evidence to recommend high-dose HD, but favor the use of a high-flux membrane.

Question

Should all patients undergoing HD 3 times weekly receive high-dose HD and use a high-flux membrane?

Answer

No, there is insufficient evidence to support the use of high-dose HD in such patients, but high-flux membranes should be used preferentially when possible.

CHAPTER 69

USE OF EPO IN CKD: THE CHOIR TRIAL

Julia Rudolf

Correction of Anemia with Epoetin Alfa in Chronic Kidney Disease

Singh AK, Szczech L, Tang KL, et al. *N Engl J Med.* 2006;355(20):2085–2098

BACKGROUND

Prior to this study, treatment with epoetin alfa had been shown to be associated with improved quality of life and reductions in cardiovascular complications and death among patients with chronic kidney disease (CKD) and anemia due to erythropoietin deficiency. However, the ideal target hemoglobin (Hgb) level was unclear given conflicting results from small interventional trials.

OBJECTIVES

To compare the effect of high- or low-target Hgb level on cardiovascular complications and death in patients with anemia due to CKD.

METHODS

Randomized, open-label trial across 130 US sites.

Patients

1,432 patients with CKD (GFR 15 to 50 mL/min/m^2). Inclusion criteria included age >18 years and Hgb <11.0 g/dL. Exclusion criteria included current dialysis, uncontrolled hypertension, active gastrointestinal bleeding, unstable angina, or a history of frequent transfusions in the preceding 6 months.

Interventions

Weekly subcutaneous epoetin alfa injections to achieve high-target Hgb level (13.5 g/dL) versus low-target level (11.3 g/dL).

Outcomes

The primary outcome was the time to the composite of death, myocardial infarction (MI), hospitalization for congestive heart failure (CHF), or stroke. Secondary outcomes included need for renal replacement therapy, and quality of life (as assessed by 3 validated scales [KDQ, SF-36, and LASA]). Serious adverse events included those that were life-threatening or resulted in hospitalization, death, or substantial disability.

KEY RESULTS

- 93.9% of patients in the low-target group (mean achieved Hgb 11.3 g/dL) and 75.9% in the high-target group (mean achieved Hgb 12.6 g/dL) had ≥1 Hgb value that reached the target.

- The incidence of the primary outcome was higher in the high-target group (17.5% vs. 13.5%, HR 1.34, 95% CI 1.03–1.74, $p = 0.03$).
- There were no statistically significant differences between the 2 groups in change from baseline quality-of-life scores except for the emotional role subset of the SF-36 quality-of-life scale (0.8 ± 48.3 in the high-target group vs. 5.9 ± 48.1 in the low-target group, $p = 0.01$).
- There was no statistically significant difference in need for renal replacement therapy (21.7% vs. 18.7%, HR 1.19, 95% CI 0.94–1.49, $p = 0.15$).
- Serious adverse events were significantly more frequent in the high-target group (54.8% vs. 48.5%, $p = 0.02$), including CHF (11.2% vs. 7.4%, $p = 0.02$).

STUDY CONCLUSIONS

A higher-target Hgb was associated with increased risk of combined death, MI, CHF, or stroke without improvement in quality of life.

COMMENTARY

CHOIR was terminated early due to the higher incidence of the composite outcome in the high-target group. Immediately prior to this study, the 2006 Kidney Disease Outcomes Quality Initiative (KDOQI) guidelines had recommended increasing the target Hgb range from 11.0–12.0 g/dL to 11.0–13.0 g/dL. Along with the simultaneously published CREATE trial,[1] which found that complete correction of anemia to Hgb 13 to 15 g/dL in CKD patients did not decrease incidence of cardiovascular events compared to partial correction to 10.5 to 11.5 g/dL, this increase was called into question. The TREAT trial[2] subsequently showed that targeting a Hgb level of 13 g/dL in diabetic CKD patients was associated with increased risk of stroke. As a result of these studies, the 2012 Kidney Disease Improving Global Outcomes clinical practice guidelines for anemia in CKD recommend treatment with erythropoietin-stimulating agents (ESAs) only if Hgb levels fall below 10 g/dL, and that they not be used to maintain Hgb levels above 11.5 g/dL.

Question

Should patients with CKD and anemia be treated with ESAs to a target Hgb level of 13.0 g/dL?

Answer

No, treatment should be considered when Hgb levels fall below 10 g/dL and should not go above 11.5 g/dL given the increased risk of adverse outcomes such as stroke and MI.

References

1. Drüeke TB, Locatelli F, Clyne N, et al. Normalization of the hemoglobin level in patients with chronic kidney disease and anemia. *N Engl J Med.* 2006;355(20):2071–2084.
2. Pfeffer MA, Burdmann EA, Chen CY, et al; TREAT Investigators. A trial of darbepoetin alfa in type 2 diabetes and chronic kidney disease. *N Engl J Med.* 2009;361(21):2019–2032.

CHAPTER 70

RENAL TRANSPLANT INDUCTION REGIMEN

Julia Rudolf

Rabbit Antithymocyte Globulin Versus Basiliximab in Renal Transplantation

Brennan DC, Daller JA, Lake KD, et al. *N Engl J Med.* 2006;355(19):1967–1977

BACKGROUND

Early in the posttransplantation period, patients are at risk for acute rejection and delayed graft function, both of which were thought to increase the risk of graft failure. At the time of this study, most patients received induction therapy with either antithymocyte globulin (ATG) or the IL-2 receptor antagonist, basiliximab, to prevent such outcomes. However, the optimal regimen was unclear particularly for patients at increased risk of acute rejection or delayed graft function.

OBJECTIVES

To compare the safety and efficacy of basiliximab and ATG in patients receiving a deceased-donor high-risk renal allograft.

METHODS

Randomized, unblinded, controlled trial in 28 US and European clinical centers between 2000 and 2002.

Patients

278 deceased-donor renal transplant recipients. Inclusion criteria included allograft features (based on donor age, donor creatinine, and absence of donor heartbeat) putting recipient at high risk for acute rejection or delayed graft function. Exclusion criteria included immunosuppressive therapy before transplant and malignancy.

Interventions

ATG (1.5 mg/kg intraoperatively, followed by daily doses through day 4) versus basiliximab (20 mg intraoperatively, followed by another dose on day 4). All patients received the same maintenance immunosuppressive therapy.

Outcomes

The primary outcome was a composite of the first occurrence of biopsy-proven acute rejection (with severe rejection defined by need for antibody treatment), delayed graft function (defined as need for dialysis within first week of transplantation), graft loss, or death. Secondary outcomes included components of the primary composite outcome and adverse events (including total events, cytopenias, infections, and cancer).

KEY RESULTS

- There were no statistically significant differences in the primary outcome (50.4% in the ATG group vs. 56.2% in the basiliximab group, $p = 0.34$).
- Fewer patients in the ATG group had biopsy-proven acute rejection (15.6% vs. 25.5%, $p = 0.02$) and severe rejection (1.4% vs. 8.0%, $p = 0.005$), but the incidence of death, delayed graft function, and graft failure were similar in both groups.
- There were no statistically significant differences in most adverse events, except for higher incidence of leukopenia (33.3% vs. 14.6%, $p < 0.001$) and infection (85.8% vs. 75.2%, $p = 0.03$) in the ATG group. There was a nonsignificant difference in the incidence of lymphoproliferative disease (3 cases in the ATG group vs. 0 in the basiliximab group, $p = 0.13$).

STUDY CONCLUSIONS

In patients at high risk for acute rejection or delayed graft function after deceased-donor kidney transplant, induction therapy with rabbit ATG reduced incidence and severity of acute rejection, but not delayed graft function or survival, compared to basiliximab.

COMMENTARY

This trial provided definitive evidence for ATG as induction therapy in high-risk patient populations in order to decrease the rate of acute rejection. A caveat is the lack of difference in graft function or graft failure between treatment groups, which may be related to the relatively short follow-up period given other studies demonstrating a link between acute rejection and graft failure. Although the ATG group exhibited increased rates of infection and lymphoproliferative disease, the benefits of ATG in reducing acute rejection are thought to outweigh the risks. This trial helped influence the 2009 Kidney Disease Improving Global Outcomes clinical practice guideline on renal allograft transplantation, which recommends ATG for induction therapy over IL-2 receptor antagonists in transplant recipients at high immunologic risk to prevent acute rejection and potentially graft failure.

Question

Should patients at high risk of rejection receive induction therapy with ATG?

Answer

Yes, compared to basiliximab, ATG leads to less acute and severe graft rejection in high-risk renal transplant patients.

ONCOLOGY

CHAPTER 71

PROSTATECTOMY VERSUS WATCHFUL WAITING FOR LOW-RISK PROSTATE CANCER: THE SPCG-4 TRIAL

Neelam A. Phadke

Radical Prostatectomy Versus Watchful Waiting in Early Prostate Cancer

Bill-Axelson A, Holmberg L, Ruutu M, et al. *N Engl J Med.* 2005;352(19):1977–1984

BACKGROUND

At the time of this study, radical prostatectomy for prostate cancer was common and appeared to reduce the risk of prostate cancer mortality. Evidence was also emerging about low-risk disease unlikely to directly affect mortality even in the setting of progression. "Watchful waiting," or treatment after development of symptoms rather than as initial curative therapy, was proposed for the management of these types of cancers. However, no long-term data about the effects of these 2 management strategies existed.

OBJECTIVES

To compare radical prostatectomy and watchful waiting in patients with low-risk prostate cancer.

METHODS

Randomized clinical trial at 14 centers in 3 Nordic countries from 1989 to 1999.

Patients

695 men. Inclusion criteria included age <75 years, new and untreated localized prostate cancer (histologically or cytologically verified with tumor stage T0d/T1b, T1, or T2/T1c), life expectancy >10 years, normal bone scan, prostate-specific antigen (PSA) level <50 ng/mL, and ability to tolerate radical prostatectomy.

Interventions

Radical prostatectomy versus watchful waiting. Transurethral resection was recommended for the treatment of urinary obstruction among men undergoing watchful waiting. Hormonal therapy was recommended for metastatic disease in all patients and for symptomatic local progression in those undergoing prostatectomy. All patients received clinical, laboratory, and radiologic monitoring.

Outcomes

The 4 main outcomes were cumulative incidence of death from prostate cancer, distant metastases, local progression, and overall mortality.

KEY RESULTS

- At 10 years, the cumulative incidence of death from prostate cancer was lower in patients receiving radical prostatectomy (RR 0.56, 95% CI 0.36–0.88, $p = 0.01$).
- The cumulative incidence of distant metastases was similar between groups at 5 years (8.1% vs. 9.8%, $p = 0.42$), but lower in those receiving prostatectomy at 10 years (15.2% vs. 25.4%, $p = 0.004$).
- At 10 years, the cumulative incidence of local progression was lower in the prostatectomy group (19.2% vs. 44.3%, $p < 0.001$).
- Overall mortality at 10 years was higher in the watchful waiting group (32.0% vs. 27.0%, $p = 0.04$).

STUDY CONCLUSIONS

Prostatectomy reduces prostate cancer-specific mortality, distant metastases, local progression, and overall mortality when compared to watchful waiting in low-risk prostate cancer.

COMMENTARY

SPCG-4 showed that "watchful waiting" was of limited utility in the majority of patients with low-risk prostate cancer and at least moderate life expectancy. Caveats include the very limited use of PSA testing to diagnose prostate cancer and possibility of missing early or small lesions. In contrast, subsequent work using PSA levels to risk stratify prostate cancer found no evidence of mortality benefit with prostatectomy over watchful waiting in lower-risk cohorts, likely delineating "very low"–risk lesions that would not have been detected otherwise.[1] As a result, the 2014 National Comprehensive Cancer Network guidelines for the management of prostate cancer recommend that patients with "very low"–risk and "low"-risk disease and >10-year life expectancy receive "active surveillance," which is distinct from "watchful waiting" and involves serial testing and curative treatment such as prostatectomy only if disease progression is found, rather than prostatectomy as initial treatment. Watchful waiting is only recommended for "very low-risk" disease in patients with <10-year life expectancy.

Question

Should patients with low-risk prostate cancer and long life expectancy be managed with "active surveillance"?

Answer

Yes, serial testing and curative treatment in the setting of disease progression are appropriate for patients with "very low"–risk and "low"-risk disease and >10-year life expectancy. In contrast, watchful waiting should be reserved for those with both "very low–risk" disease and shorter life expectancy.

References

1. Wilt TJ, Brawer MK, Jones KM, et al. Radical prostatectomy versus observation for localized prostate cancer. *N Engl J Med.* 2012;367(3):203–213.

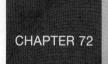

| CHAPTER 72 | LOW-DOSE CT FOR LUNG CANCER SCREENING: THE NLST |

Neelam A. Phadke

Reduced Lung-Cancer Mortality With Low-Dose Computed Tomographic Screening
Aberle DR, Adams AM, Berg CD, et al. *N Engl J Med.* 2011;365(5):395–409

BACKGROUND

Prior studies had failed to demonstrate a reduction in lung cancer mortality with chest x-ray (CXR) screening. In turn, observational studies, however, showed that low-dose helical lung computed tomography (LDCT) exposed patients to acceptable levels of radiation while detecting more lung nodules and cancers compared to CXR.

OBJECTIVES

To determine if LDCT screening of high-risk persons could reduce lung cancer mortality.

METHODS

Randomized controlled trial in 33 US medical centers with enrollment from 2002 to 2004.

Patients

53,454 patients. Inclusion criteria included age 55 to 74 years, ≥30 pack-year smoking history, and if former smokers, quit date within the previous 15 years. Exclusion criteria included prior lung cancer diagnosis, chest CT within 18 months prior to enrollment, hemoptysis, or unexplained weight loss (>6.8 kg in past year).

Interventions

LDCT versus CXR. All patients were eligible for up to 3 annual standard protocol studies (or until lung cancer detected), which were reviewed by specially trained radiologists, both in isolation and in the context of historical images. A CT scan with any noncalcified nodule ≥4 mm in any diameter or a CXR with any noncalcified nodule or mass was considered positive (i.e., concerning for malignancy). Adenopathy, effusion, and other abnormalities could also be classified as positive. The median follow-up was 6.5 years.

Outcomes

The primary outcome was difference in lung cancer mortality (per 100,000 person years) between LDCT and CXR. Secondary outcomes included the rate of death from any cause and incidence of lung cancer.

KEY RESULTS

- There were fewer lung cancer deaths in the LDCT group (247 vs. 309 per 100,000 person years, relative risk reduction 20.0%, 95% CI, 6.8%–26.7%, $p = 0.004$).
- There were fewer deaths from any cause in the LDCT group (1,877 vs. 2,000, relative risk reduction 6.7%, 95% CI, 1.2%–13.6%, $p = 0.02$).
- More patients undergoing LDCT had ≥1 positive screening result (39.1% vs. 16.0%, no p value reported).
- Among patients who underwent diagnostic evaluation after a positive screening result, the rate of at least one complication was low (1.4% in the LDCT group vs. 1.6% in the CXR group).

STUDY CONCLUSIONS

LDCT reduces lung cancer mortality when compared to CXR.

COMMENTARY

This study proved that LDCT for lung cancer screening reduced mortality in current and former smokers. It is important to note that LDCT carried a risk of false positives; however, diagnostic CT and review of previous imaging led to few invasive diagnostic procedures. Caveats include the role of the "healthy-volunteer" effect and the rigorous radiologist training protocol in the study, which may not have been representative of standard care. Questions remain regarding screening frequency and duration as well as cost-effectiveness relative to other interventions such as smoking cessation counseling and screening with molecular markers. A follow-up study demonstrated a cost of $81,000 per quality-adjusted life-year for LDCT screening, with highest cost-effectiveness among women, current smokers, and older groups.[1] Given the compelling mortality benefit, this study directly led to the 2014 US Preventive Services Task Force lung cancer screening update recommending LDCT in high-risk populations.

Question

Should patients at high risk for lung cancer undergo LDCT screening?

Answer

Yes, screening with LDCT reduces mortality when compared to CXR.

References

1. Black WC, Gareen IF, Soneji SS. Cost-effectiveness of CT screening in the National Lung Screening Trial. *N Engl J Med.* 2014;371(19):1793–1802.

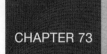

CHAPTER 73

OXALIPLATIN AS ADJUVANT THERAPY IN COLON CANCER: THE MOSAIC TRIAL

Daniel O'Neil

Oxaliplatin, Fluorouracil, and Leucovorin as Adjuvant Treatment for Colon Cancer
André T, Boni C, Mounedji-Boudiaf L, et al. *N Engl J Med.* 2004;350(23):2343–2351

BACKGROUND

In the 1990s, fluorouracil plus leucovorin (FL) chemotherapy represented a standard adjuvant therapy for colon cancer. Oxaliplatin, a third-generation platinum derivative, had also been shown to be efficacious for treatment of metastatic colorectal cancer. The benefit of adding oxaliplatin to adjuvant FL (FOLFOX) in earlier stage disease was unknown.

OBJECTIVES

To determine if the addition of oxaliplatin to FL benefits patients with stage II and III colon cancer.

METHODS

Randomized, open-label trial at 146 centers in 20 countries in Europe, Australia, and Asia from 1998 to 2001.

Patients

2,246 patients. Inclusion criteria included histologically diagnosed stage II or III colon cancer with complete resection, age 18 to 75 years, and good performance status (Karnofsky performance status score ≥60). Exclusion criteria included prior chemotherapy or radiotherapy.

Intervention

FOLFOX versus FL. Median follow-up was 37.9 months.

Outcomes

The primary efficacy outcome was disease-free survival (DFS) at 3 years, with relapse defined by imaging or cytologic analysis or biopsy. DFS was also analyzed by groups based on stage of disease, age, and other variables. Other secondary outcomes included overall survival (OS) and adverse reactions (including severe neuropathy and neutropenia, with and without infection).

KEY RESULTS

- DFS was improved in the FOLFOX group (HR 0.77, 95% CI 0.65–0.91, p = 0.002).
- FOLFOX was associated with improved DFS in stage III patients (HR 0.76, 95% CI 0.62–0.92) but not in stage II patients (HR 0.80, 95% CI 0.56–1.15).

- OS was not statistically significantly different between the total FOLFOX and FL groups (HR 0.90, 95% CI 0.71–1.13).
- Rates of severe neuropathy (12.4% vs. 0.2%, $p = 0.001$), and neutropenia with infection (1.8% vs. 0.2%, $p < 0.001$) were higher in the FOLFOX group.

STUDY CONCLUSIONS

The addition of oxaliplatin to FL improves adjuvant treatment of colon cancer.

COMMENTARY

MOSAIC established oxaliplatin as an important adjuvant therapy for stage III colon cancer. Caveats include what some thought was a short follow-up time. Indeed, longer follow-up eventually demonstrated improvement in OS in the entire group, although subgroup analysis showed no benefit for FOLFOX in stage II disease or in patients >70 years old. Thus, the entire benefit was driven by stage III patients, particularly those with the most advanced disease. These findings are particularly important given the high rates of adverse events associated with oxaliplatin, which include irreversible neuropathy and liver damage. Considering the current evidence, the 2016 National Comprehensive Cancer Network guidelines endorse FOLFOX adjuvant chemotherapy only in stage III patients <70 years old.

Question

Should younger patients with stage III colon cancer receive adjuvant oxaliplatin in addition to FL?

Answer

Yes, adjuvant oxaliplatin yields an independent survival benefit in these cases.

CHAPTER 74

EGFR INHIBITION IN NON–SMALL-CELL LUNG CANCER: THE IPASS TRIAL

Mounica Vallurupalli

Gefitinib or Carboplatin-Paclitaxel in Pulmonary Adenocarcinoma

Mok TS, Wu YL, Thongprasert S, et al. *N Engl J Med.* 2009;361(10):947–957

BACKGROUND

The epidermal growth factor receptor (EGFR) is a tyrosine kinase that can be mutated in non–small-cell lung cancer (NSCLC), resulting in increased receptor activity and stimulation of tumor cell growth. Prior to this study, EGFR tyrosine-kinase inhibitors (TKIs) had been associated with dramatic benefit among patients with tumors harboring activating EGFR mutations (most commonly never/light smokers, women, and Asians). However, head-to-head comparisons of an EGFR TKI and standard chemotherapy as first-line treatment in advanced NSCLC were lacking.

OBJECTIVES

To compare the effectiveness of gefitinib, an oral EGFR TKI, to standard cytotoxic chemotherapy as initial treatment of advanced lung adenocarcinoma.

METHODS

Randomized, open-label, controlled noninferiority trial in 87 centers in East Asia between 2006 and 2007.

Patients

1,217 patients. Inclusion criteria included age ≥18 years, nonsmoker (<100 lifetime cigarettes) or light smoker (≤10 pack-years with ≥15 years of smoking cessation) status, and histologically or cytologically proven stage IIIB or IV NSCLC (with adenocarcinoma features), and no prior chemotherapy. Planned subgroup analyses included those based on the presence or absence of an activating EGFR mutation.

Interventions

Gefitinib (250 mg daily) versus carboplatin–paclitaxel chemotherapy. Treatment was administered until completion of 6 cycles of chemotherapy, progression of disease, unacceptable toxic effects, protocol noncompliance, or request by the patient or physician to discontinue therapy.

Outcomes

The primary outcome was progression-free survival (PFS). Other outcomes included overall survival (OS) and quality of life.

KEY RESULTS

- Overall PFS at 12 months was greater in the gefitinib group (24.9% vs. 6.7%, HR 0.74, 95% CI 0.65–0.85, $p < 0.001$).
- Among the 261 EGFR mutation-positive patients, PFS was longer in those receiving gefitinib (HR 0.48, 95% CI 0.36–0.64, $p < 0.001$).
- Among the 176 EGFR mutation-negative patients, PFS was longer in those receiving carboplatin–paclitaxel (HR 2.85, 95% CI 2.05–3.98, $p < 0.001$).
- There was no statistically significant difference in OS (HR 0.91, 95% CI 0.76–1.10).
- The gefitinib group experienced lower rates of severe or life-threatening adverse effects (28.7% vs. 61.0%) and adverse events resulting in therapy discontinuation (6.9% vs. 13.6%).

STUDY CONCLUSIONS

Gefitinib is superior to carboplatin–paclitaxel as first-line treatment of lung adenocarcinoma among light- and nonsmokers from East Asia.

COMMENTARY

IPASS was the first randomized trial to demonstrate the superiority of targeted therapy in NSCLC when matched to a genetic biomarker. Its main finding – that the presence of an activating EGFR mutation strongly predicts better outcomes with EGFR TKIs compared to cytotoxic chemotherapy – has been confirmed by subsequent studies excluding patients with wild-type EGFR genes. To date, several EGFR TKIs (erlotinib, gefitinib, and afatinib) are approved for first-line treatment of EGFR-mutant NSCLC, with next-generation TKIs used to treat resistance to first-line agents. More broadly, this approach is emblematic of the move toward precision cancer care, with treatment decisions increasingly guided by tumor genomics. The 2016 National Comprehensive Cancer Network lung cancer treatment guidelines recommend routine testing for several key oncogenic mutations in patients with lung adenocarcinoma and initiation of targeted therapy as first-line therapy if such a mutation is present.

Question

Should patients with NSCLC and an activating EGFR mutation receive an EGFR inhibitor as first-line therapy?

Answer

Yes, first-line EGFR TKIs are superior to standard cytotoxic therapy in patients with activating EGFR mutations.

CHAPTER 75

HER2-TARGETED THERAPY IN BREAST CANCER

Erik H. Knelson

Use of Chemotherapy Plus a Monoclonal Antibody Against HER2 for Metastatic Breast Cancer That Overexpresses HER2

Slamon DJ, Leyland-Jones B, Shak S, et al. *N Engl J Med*. 2001;344(11):783–792

BACKGROUND

Prior to 2001, there were no specific treatments beyond standard therapy for human epidermal growth factor receptor-2 (HER2)-amplified breast cancer, an aggressive variant representing 25% to 30% of cases. The humanized HER2 monoclonal antibody trastuzumab, one of the first molecularly targeted therapies in oncology, proved safe in preliminary trials of women with pretreated metastatic HER2-amplified breast cancer, leading to this larger study.

OBJECTIVES

To determine whether the addition of trastuzumab to standard chemotherapy could increase clinical benefit in metastatic HER2-amplified breast cancer.

METHODS

Randomized, double-blind, controlled trial between 1995 and 1997.

Patients

469 patients. Inclusion criteria included progressive metastatic HER2-amplified breast cancer without receipt of chemotherapy for metastatic disease. Exclusion criteria included bilateral breast cancer, untreated brain metastasis or osteoblastic bone metastasis, poor performance status (Karnofsky score <60), pregnancy, or second malignancy.

Intervention

Trastuzumab plus chemotherapy versus chemotherapy alone. Standard chemotherapy included an anthracycline plus cyclophosphamide, or paclitaxel alone if previously treated with an anthracycline.

Outcomes

The primary outcome was time to disease progression, defined as an increase of >25% in the dimensions of any measurable lesion. Secondary outcomes included rate of objective response, response duration, time to treatment failure (composite of death, disease progression, treatment discontinuation, and use of other types of antitumor therapy), survival, and adverse events.

KEY RESULTS

- Median time to disease progression was longer in the trastuzumab group (7.4 months vs. 4.6 months, $p < 0.001$), regardless of the chemotherapeutic regimen used.
- Patients receiving trastuzumab had a lower 1-year death rate (22% vs. 33%, $p = 0.008$), and longer median survival (25.1 months vs. 20.3 months, $p = 0.046$).
- Trastuzumab was associated with a higher rate of overall response (50% vs. 32%, $p < 0.001$), longer median duration of response (9.1 months vs. 6.1 months, $p < 0.001$), and a longer time to treatment failure (median 6.9 months vs. 4.5 months, $p < 0.001$) regardless of the chemotherapeutic regimen used.
- Trastuzumab increased cardiac dysfunction (with or without symptoms) when added to chemotherapy (27% in combination with doxorubicin/cyclophosphamide and 13% in combination with paclitaxel vs. 8% and 1% with these chemotherapy regimens alone, no p values reported).

STUDY CONCLUSIONS

Trastuzumab lengthened the time to disease progression and improved therapeutic response in women with metastatic HER2-amplified breast cancer.

COMMENTARY

This trial established the use of first-line trastuzumab in combination with chemotherapy for women with metastatic HER2-amplified breast cancer and led to prompt FDA approval for this indication primarily given the improvement in survival associated with its use. Importantly, the cardiac toxicities documented in this trial were subsequently found to be reversible after cessation of therapy. Based on subsequent work,[1] trastuzumab's indications were expanded to include adjuvant treatment of early-stage HER2-amplified breast cancers. More generally, trastuzumab informed the development of other molecularly targeted cancer therapies and therapeutic monoclonal antibodies. Guidelines from the American Society of Clinical Oncology now recommend HER2-targeted therapy in the vast majority of patients with HER2-positive breast cancer.

Question

Should women with HER2-amplified breast cancer receive a HER2-targeted therapy as part of treatment?

Answer

Yes, the addition of HER2 inhibitors to chemotherapy improves survival, although it also increases the risk of cardiotoxicity.

References

1. Piccart-Gebhart MJ, Procter M, Leyland-Jones B, et al; Herceptin Adjuvant (HERA) Trial Study Team. Trastuzumab after adjuvant chemotherapy in HER2-positive breast cancer. *N Engl J Med.* 2005;353:1659–1672.

CHAPTER 76

POLYPECTOMY TO PREVENT COLORECTAL CANCER: THE NATIONAL POLYP STUDY

Daniel O'Neil

Prevention of Colorectal Cancer by Colonoscopic Polypectomy

Winawer SJ, Zauber AG, Ho MN, et al. *N Engl J Med*. 1993;329(27):1977–1981

BACKGROUND

In the 1970s, adenomatous polyps were recognized as precursors to colorectal cancer (CRC). The advent of fiberoptic colonoscopy enabled the endoscopic removal of these lesions with the intent to prevent CRC, but efficacy data validating this practice were lacking. The National Polyp Study (NPS) was designed to determine the best follow-up approach after polypectomy, randomizing patients to varying intervals for repeat colonoscopy. However, it also generated a large dataset of postpolypectomy patients, which allowed for prospective examination of CRC risk.

OBJECTIVES

To determine if colonoscopic polypectomy reduces the incidence of CRC.

METHODS

Observational study of the cohort from the NPS, which was conducted at 7 sites in the United States from 1980 to 1990, compared to 3 historical reference cohorts.

Patients

1,379 patients from the NPS who underwent colonoscopic polypectomy and were not lost to follow up. NPS excluded patients prior to colonoscopic polypectomy with a history of previous polypectomy, CRC, or familial polyposis, as well as after colonoscopic polypectomy if it revealed malignancy, nonadenomatous polyps, large sessile polyps, or no polyps. The reference cohorts were: 226 Mayo Clinic patients from 1965 to 1970 with polyps ≥1 cm that declined surgical polypectomy; 1,618 St. Mark's Hospital patients from 1957 to 1980 undergoing rectosigmoid polypectomy without distal colon examination; and a 10% sample from the standard risk population in the Surveillance, Epidemiology, and End Results (SEER) database from 1983 to 1987.

Intervention

Retrospective comparison of observed and expected CRC incidence rates. In the NPS, all patients completed colonoscopic polypectomy. Mean follow-up was 5.9 years.

Outcomes

The primary outcome was standardized incidence ratio (SIR), which was calculated by comparing the observed incidence of CRC in the NPS cohort with that derived from each of the reference cohorts. Ratios <1 indicated a lower than expected incidence in the NPS cohort. Secondary outcomes included subgroup analyses of patients with large (>1 cm) and small (≤1 cm) adenomas.

KEY RESULTS

- 5 cases of CRC were detected in the NPS cohort, compared with 48.3 expected based on the Mayo cohort (SIR = 0.1, 95% CI 0.03–0.24, $p < 0.001$), 43.4 expected based on the St. Mark's cohort (SIR = 0.12, 95% CI 0.04–0.27, $p < 0.001$), and 20.7 expected based on the SEER cohort (SIR = 0.24, 95% CI 0.08–0.56, $p < 0.001$).
- 3 cases of CRC were detected in NPS patients with large adenomas, compared with 40.2 expected based on the Mayo cohort (SIR 0.07, 95% CI 0.02–0.22).

STUDY CONCLUSIONS

Colonoscopic polypectomy in patients with adenomas reduces the incidence of CRC when compared to the general population and cohorts of patients with polyps.

COMMENTARY

This analysis of NLP was one of the first to show that as part of endoscopic surveillance, polypectomy reduced the incidence of CRC to a level below even that of an average-risk population (as defined by the SEER cohort), and extended follow-up of these patients subsequently revealed a mortality benefit. Even though less invasive techniques have since been developed to detect CRC itself, rather than precancerous polyps, the lack of evidence regarding follow-up intervals and a high rate of false-positive results have precluded these methods from supplanting polypectomy as standard of care for CRC prevention. The 2012 American College of Gastroenterology colonoscopy surveillance guidelines endorse polypectomy as the definitive preventive strategy against CRC.

Question

Should patients receive polypectomy during colonoscopy to reduce CRC incidence?

Answer

Yes, polypectomy reduces CRC incidence and mortality as a method of primary cancer prevention.

CHAPTER 77

PREVENTION OF RECURRENT VTE WITH LMWH IN PATIENTS WITH CANCER: THE CLOT TRIAL

Neelam A. Phadke

Low-Molecular-Weight Heparin Versus a Coumarin for the Prevention of Recurrent Venous Thromboembolism in Patients With Cancer

Lee AYY, Levine MN, Baker RI, et al. *N Engl J Med.* 2003;349(2):146–153

BACKGROUND

At the time of this study, low–molecular-weight heparin (LMWH) or unfractionated heparin, followed by long-term oral anticoagulation with a vitamin K antagonist, represented standard therapy for acute venous thromboembolism (VTE). Given more predictable pharmacokinetics, fewer drug interactions, reduced need for drug level monitoring, and decreased concern for missed doses due to nausea, LMWHs were hypothesized to be potentially more effective and practical for anticoagulation among cancer patients at increased risk for recurrent thrombosis.

OBJECTIVES

To investigate whether the LMWH dalteparin is safer and more effective than oral vitamin K antagonist therapy in preventing recurrent VTE in cancer patients.

METHODS

Randomized, open-label, controlled trial across 48 clinical centers in 8 countries in North America, Europe, and Australia from 1999 to 2001.

Patients

676 patients. Inclusion criteria included active cancer and newly diagnosed, symptomatic VTE (pulmonary embolism and/or proximal deep venous thrombosis). Exclusion criteria included weight <40 kg, poor performance status (Eastern Cooperative Oncology Group score 3 or 4), heparin treatment for >48 hours before randomization, current oral anticoagulation, elevated creatinine, recent serious bleeding, or high risk of serious bleeding (including thrombocytopenia).

Interventions

Dalteparin (200 IU/kg daily subcutaneous injection for 1 month followed by ~150 IU/kg for 5 months) versus a vitamin K antagonist (titrated with a 5 to 7-day dalteparin bridge to a goal INR 2.0 to 3.0 for 6 months).

Outcomes

The primary outcome was the first episode of objectively documented, symptomatic, recurrent VTE. Secondary outcomes included clinically overt bleeding (defined as major or any) and death.

KEY RESULTS

- Symptomatic, recurrent VTE occurred in fewer patients in the dalteparin group (8.0% vs. 15.8%, HR 0.48, 95% CI 0.30–0.77, p = 0.002).
- There were no significant differences in the rate of major bleeding (6% vs. 4% favoring oral anticoagulant, p = 0.27) or any bleeding (14% vs. 19% favoring dalteparin, p = 0.09).
- There was no statistically significant difference in mortality rates at 6 months (39% in the dalteparin group vs. 41% in the oral anticoagulation group, p = 0.53). 90% of deaths in both groups were due to cancer progression.

STUDY CONCLUSIONS

Compared to oral vitamin K antagonists, dalteparin reduces the occurrence of symptomatic, recurrent VTE without significantly increasing bleeding risk among patients with active cancer.

COMMENTARY

The CLOT trial directly influenced the standard of care in cancer patients presenting with VTE. While the study's open-label design and drug-company sponsorship were recognized as weaknesses, the use of objective outcome tests with blinded adjudication mitigated these effects. Also notable is the short duration of follow-up in this study. Importantly, these results are not generalizable to the direct oral anticoagulants (DOACs), and head-to-head comparisons between LMWH and DOACs are ongoing. As a result of this trial, the 2007 American Society of Clinical Oncology recommends LMWH as monotherapy for malignancy-associated VTE, to be continued indefinitely unless the cancer is cured or it is unsafe to do so.

Question

Should patients with VTE and active cancer receive LMWH instead of oral vitamin K antagonists?

Answer

Yes, LMWH is superior in reducing the risk of symptomatic, recurrent VTE without increasing the risk of bleeding.

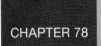

BREAST-CONSERVING SURGERY FOR EARLY BREAST CANCER

CHAPTER 78

Erik H. Knelson

Twenty-Year Follow-Up of a Randomized Study Comparing Breast-Conserving Surgery With Radical Mastectomy for Early Breast Cancer

Veronesi U, Cascinelli N, Mariani L, et al. *N Engl J Med*. 2002;347(16):1227–1232

BACKGROUND

In the 1970s, surgeons and patients doubted whether radical mastectomy, a disfiguring operation, was necessary given new developments in radiotherapy, chemotherapy, and surgical techniques. Comparison trials began enrolling around that time, and preliminary results in the late 1970s and early 1980s demonstrated no difference in survival between radical mastectomy and breast-conserving therapy (BCT) sparing muscle and breast tissue. Given the short follow-up for these trials and the extended latency of recurrence for small tumors, questions lingered regarding the equivalency in outcomes with BCT.

OBJECTIVES

To compare long-term outcomes after radical mastectomy or BCT in women with small, localized breast cancers.

METHODS

Randomized controlled trial at a single Italian center between 1973 and 1980.

Patients

701 women. Inclusion criteria included T1N0 infiltrating breast carcinoma (defined as ≤2 cm and without palpable axillary lymph nodes on physical examination). Exclusion criteria included age >70 years and previous cancer.

Interventions

BCT (quadrantectomy, complete axillary node dissection, and radiotherapy) versus radical mastectomy. Beginning in 1976, all patients in both groups with axillary lymph node disease found after node dissection received 12 months of adjuvant chemotherapy (cyclophosphamide, methotrexate, and fluorouracil).

Outcomes

Outcomes included overall survival (OS), mortality from breast cancer, local recurrence (defined as ipsilateral breast cancer recurrence), distant metastasis, contralateral breast cancer, and second primary cancer.

KEY RESULTS

- OS at 20 years was similar in both groups (41.2% mortality following radical mastectomy vs. 41.7% with BCT, $p = 1.0$).
- Mortality from breast cancer was similar in both groups (24.3% with radical mastectomy vs. 26.1% following BCT, $p = 0.8$).
- Incidence of local recurrence was higher with BCT (8.8% vs. 2.3%, $p < 0.001$).
- There were no statistically significant differences in rates of contralateral recurrence, distant metastasis, or other primary cancers.

STUDY CONCLUSIONS

Treatment of early-stage breast cancer with BCT or radical mastectomy leads to similar long-term survival.

COMMENTARY

This pivotal trial reaffirmed earlier findings from the same cohort after an impressive 20-year prospective follow-up period, and, alongside a similar trial in the United States,[1] confirmed the equivalence in clinical outcomes between BCT and radical mastectomy. It is important to note that although the risk of recurrence in the same breast was higher with BCT, only 10 of these tumors were along the scar from the previous resection and thus ostensibly true recurrences. The remaining 20 tumors likely represented new cancers, highlighting the increased risk of women with a prior diagnosis of breast cancer rather than failure of BCT. Important caveats include that hormone receptor status was not assessed and hormonal therapies were not employed. Overall, this trial exemplifies the subsequent trend toward less invasive approaches in the treatment of early-stage breast cancer. Today, quadrantectomy and axillary lymph node dissection have been supplanted in most cases by lumpectomy with sentinel node biopsy and a greater focus on the treatment of micrometastatic disease with adjuvant systemic therapy. The 2015 guidelines from the American Society of Breast Surgeons recommend BCT in most cases of early-stage breast cancer.

Question

Should women with early-stage breast cancer undergo radical mastectomy?

Answer

No, radical mastectomy offers no survival benefit over BCT, which has become increasingly less invasive over time.

References

1. Fisher B, Jeong JH, Anderson S, Bryant J, Fisher ER, Wolmark N. Twenty-five-year follow-up of a randomized trial comparing radical mastectomy, total mastectomy, and total mastectomy followed by irradiation. *N Engl J Med.* 2002;347(8):567–575.

CHAPTER 79

BEVACIZUMAB IN METASTATIC COLORECTAL CANCER TREATMENT

Daniel O'Neil

Bevacizumab Plus Irinotecan, Fluorouracil, and Leucovorin for Metastatic Colorectal Cancer

Hurwitz H, Fehrenbacher L, Novotny W, et al. *N Engl J Med*. 2004;350(23):2335–2342

BACKGROUND

Bevacizumab, a monoclonal antibody directed against the vascular endothelial growth factor, was hypothesized to interfere with tumor angiogenesis and increase chemotherapy uptake in cancer cells. Although a phase 2 trial suggested that bevacizumab improved survival in metastatic colorectal cancer when added to standard chemotherapy, a definitive clinical trial to assess its efficacy was warranted.

OBJECTIVES

To determine if the addition of bevacizumab improves survival among patients with metastatic colorectal cancer when added to irinotecan, fluorouracil, and leucovorin (IFL) chemotherapy.

METHODS

Randomized, placebo-controlled trial at 164 sites in the United States, Australia, and New Zealand between 2000 and 2002.

Patients

813 patients. Inclusion criteria included age ≥18 years, metastatic colorectal cancer, excellent performance status (Eastern Cooperative Oncology Group score of 0 or 1), and adequate hematologic, hepatic, and renal function. Exclusion criteria included prior systemic therapy for metastatic disease within 12 months and recent radiotherapy or surgery.

Intervention

IFL plus bevacizumab versus IFL plus placebo every 2 weeks. (A third arm, FL plus bevacizumab, was halted after an interim analysis demonstrated an acceptable safety profile for bevacizumab plus IFL.) These treatments continued for 96 weeks or until disease progression or intolerable toxicity.

Outcomes

The primary outcome was overall survival (OS). Secondary outcomes included progression-free survival (PFS), partial and complete response rates, duration of response, and adverse reactions (including those leading to hospitalization and the incidence of hypertension, leukopenia, and diarrhea).

KEY RESULTS

- Median OS was greater in patients who received bevacizumab (20.3 months vs. 15.6 months, HR = 0.66, $p < 0.001$).
- Median PFS was longer in the bevacizumab group (10.6 months vs. 6.2 months, HR = 0.54, $p < 0.001$).
- Hypertension was more frequent in the bevacizumab group (22.4% vs. 8.3%, $p < 0.01$).
- There were no statistically significant differences in severe or life-threatening leukopenia (37.0% vs. 31.1%), severe or life-threatening diarrhea (32.4% vs. 24.7%), or adverse events leading to hospitalization (44.9% vs. 39.6%) between the bevacizumab and placebo groups, respectively.

STUDY CONCLUSIONS

The addition of bevacizumab to IFL improves OS and PFS in metastatic colorectal cancer.

COMMENTARY

This study was the first to show that bevacizumab prolongs OS when added to one of the most commonly used regimens for metastatic colorectal cancer. Caveats include unclear mechanism of benefit (since bevacizumab targets angiogenesis and colorectal cancer is hypovascular) and study completion before other beneficial treatments, such as oxaliplatin, were widely available and used. Later work demonstrated a survival benefit with the addition of bevacizumab to other chemotherapy-based regimens, although not as part of adjuvant therapy.[1,2] As a result, the 2015 National Comprehensive Cancer Network guidelines on colorectal cancer treatment recommend bevacizumab as a potential adjunctive agent for first-line therapy in metastatic disease.

Question

Is it reasonable to treat patients with metastatic colorectal cancer with bevacizumab?

Answer

Yes, when added to standard chemotherapy, bevacizumab improves survival in metastatic disease.

References

1. Cao Y, Tan A, Gao F, Liu L, Liao C, Mo Z. A meta-analysis of randomized controlled trials comparing chemotherapy plus bevacizumab with chemotherapy alone in metastatic colorectal cancer. *Int J Colorectal Dis.* 2009;24(6):677–685.
2. Allegra CJ, Yothers G, O'Connell MJ, et al. Bevacizumab in stage II-III colon cancer: 5-year update of the National Surgical Adjuvant Breast and Bowel Project C-08 trial. *J Clin Oncol.* 2013;31(3):359–364.

CHAPTER 80

AROMATASE INHIBITORS IN EARLY BREAST CANCER

Mounica Vallurupalli

A Comparison of Letrozole and Tamoxifen in Postmenopausal Women With Early Breast Cancer

Thürlimann B, Keshaviah A, Coates AS, et al. *N Engl J Med.* 2005;353(26):2747–2757

BACKGROUND

Prior to this trial, tamoxifen therapy was known to improve outcomes in early breast cancer but increase the risk of thromboembolism and endometrial cancer. After aromatase inhibitors (AIs) such as letrozole were found to be equivalent or superior to tamoxifen for hormone-receptor-positive (HR+) metastatic breast cancer, salvage AI therapy became a mainstay of treatment. Despite other studies supporting AIs in earlier-stage disease, either over tamoxifen as primary adjuvant therapy or in sequence following 2 to 3 years of adjuvant tamoxifen, a definitive trial was needed.

OBJECTIVES

To compare the efficacy and risks of AIs versus tamoxifen in early-stage HR+ breast cancer.

METHODS

Randomized, double-blind controlled international trial from 1998 to 2003.

Patients

8,010 postmenopausal women with breast cancer. Inclusion criteria included HR positivity (estrogen, progesterone, or both) and clear margins after primary surgery. Exclusion criteria included evidence of metastatic disease and previous adjuvant therapy use.

Interventions

Letrozole (2.5 mg daily) versus tamoxifen (20 mg daily). These groups consisted of patients randomized to 4 administration arms: those receiving letrozole or tamoxifen monotherapy (for 5 years), and those receiving sequential permutations of tamoxifen and letrozole (the first medication given for 2 years and included in this analysis; the second for 3 years and excluded from this analysis). Median follow-up was 25.8 months.

Outcomes

The primary outcome was disease-free survival (DFS), which included development of any second, nonbreast cancer. Secondary outcomes included overall survival (OS), systemic DFS, the occurrence of a nonbreast cancer, time to distant recurrence, and safety (venous thromboembolism, endometrial cancer, vaginal bleeding, fracture risk, and others).

KEY RESULTS

- DFS was higher at 5 years in the letrozole group (84.0% vs. 81.4%, HR 0.81, 95% CI 0.70–0.93, $p = 0.003$).
- There was no statistically significant difference in OS (166 died in the letrozole group vs. 192 in the tamoxifen group, HR 0.86, 95% CI 0.70–1.06, $p = 0.16$).
- The risk of distant recurrence was lower in those receiving letrozole (HR 0.73, 95% CI 0.60–0.88, $p = 0.001$).
- Women receiving tamoxifen were more likely to develop venous thromboembolism (3.5% vs. 1.5%, $p < 0.001$), invasive endometrial cancer (0.3% vs. 0.1%, $p = 0.18$), and vaginal bleeding (6.6% vs. 3.3%, $p < 0.001$) while those treated with letrozole experienced more fractures (5.7% vs. 4.0%, $p < 0.001$).

STUDY CONCLUSIONS

Letrozole is safe and more effective than tamoxifen as adjuvant treatment in early-stage HR+ breast cancer in postmenopausal women.

COMMENTARY

After this study, AIs became part of the standard treatment of early-stage HR+ breast cancer in postmenopausal women. Moreover, this trial provided data about the distinct safety profiles of AIs and tamoxifen, further guiding their use. A limitation of this study was the relatively short follow-up time in which to detect differences in mortality. Longer-term analysis of this trial[1] confirmed greater DFS and no difference in OS for letrozole monotherapy compared to tamoxifen monotherapy at 5 years, while also demonstrating no difference in OS or DFS between 5 years of letrozole and either of the 2 sequential permutation arms. The results of these studies led to an update of the 2007 National Comprehensive Cancer Network guidelines, which now recommend the use of AIs over tamoxifen for early-stage HR+ breast cancer in postmenopausal women.

Question

Should postmenopausal women receive AIs as adjuvant therapy for early-stage HR+ breast cancer?

Answer

Yes, AI therapy offers greater DFS and a better safety profile than tamoxifen.

References

1. Mouridsen H, Giobbie-Hurder A, Goldhirsch A, et al; BIG 1–98 Collaborative Group. Letrozole therapy alone or in sequence with tamoxifen in women with breast cancer. *N Engl J Med.* 2009;361(8):766–776.

PULMONOLOGY

CHAPTER 81

THE WELLS SCORE FOR PULMONARY EMBOLISM

Elizabeth A. Richey

Excluding Pulmonary Embolism at the Bedside Without Diagnostic Imaging: Management of Patients With Suspected Pulmonary Embolism Presenting to the Emergency Department by Using a Simple Clinical Model and D-dimer

Wells PS, Anderson DR, Rodger M, et al. *Ann Intern Med.* 2001;135(2):98–107

BACKGROUND

The nonspecific signs and symptoms associated with pulmonary embolism (PE) pose diagnostic dilemmas: poor access to imaging can cause diagnostic delays while overuse can produce unnecessary harms for those without PE. Despite prior attempts to use diagnostic algorithms to identify the appropriate patients to test, their utility in the emergency department (ED) setting remained unknown.

OBJECTIVES

To evaluate the safety of a diagnostic algorithm that combines a clinical decision tool with serum D-dimer measurement to manage patients with suspected PE.

METHODS

Prospective cohort study from 4 Canadian tertiary care hospitals between 1998 and 1999.

Patients

930 adults presenting to the ED with symptoms suggestive of PE (acute onset or worsening shortness of breath or chest pain). Exclusion criteria included pregnancy, life expectancy <3 months, anticoagulation for >24 hours, and contraindication to intravenous contrast.

Interventions

The following decision tool was applied to all patients to determine the clinical probability of PE.

Variable	Points
Clinical signs and symptoms of DVT, PE as likely as or more likely than alternative diagnosis	3.0 each
HR >100, prior venous thromboembolism, immobilization for ≥3 days or surgery in the previous 4 weeks	1.5 each
Hemoptysis, malignancy	1.0 each

Score
Low probability   <2
Intermediate probability   2–6
High probability   >6

D-dimer testing was also performed in all patients after applying the tool. PE was considered excluded among patients with negative D-dimer tests *and* deemed to have low clinical probability of disease. All others underwent diagnostic imaging with ventilation–perfusion lung scanning.

Outcomes

The primary outcome was the proportion of patients with a venous thromboembolic (VTE) event during 3 months of follow-up among those who had PE excluded via the algorithm.

KEY RESULTS

- The clinical decision tool classified 7% of patients with high probability, 36% with moderate probability, and 57% with low probability of having PE.
- Of the 759 patients in whom PE was considered excluded, 0.1% (95% CI 0.0%–0.7%) developed a VTE event during follow-up.
- The negative predictive value of the algorithm ranged from 99.5% (95% CI 99.1%–100%) in patients with low clinical probability to 88.5% (95% CI 69.9%–97.6%) in those with high clinical probability.

STUDY CONCLUSIONS

Managing patients for suspected PE based on pretest probability and the results of D-dimer testing is safe and decreases the need for diagnostic imaging.

COMMENTARY

This study was the first to describe a reliable clinical decision tool (which came to be known as the "Wells score") that continues to be used in multiple settings to guide the evaluation of suspected PE. Notably, the score relies on subjective clinical assessment and was originally paired with ventilation–perfusion scanning instead of other contemporary imaging modalities. The criteria have since been adapted and validated in other settings and circumstances (e.g., into a dichotomized score using CT angiography). Based on this collective evidence, the 2015 American College of Physicians PE guidelines recommend the use of the Wells score or another stratification tool to evaluate suspected PE.

Question

Should patients with a negative D-dimer and a Wells score of 1 undergo diagnostic imaging for suspected PE?

Answer

No, the diagnosis can be safely excluded in nearly all patients with low clinical probability of PE (Wells score <2) and negative D-dimer, though other tools can also be used to estimate pretest probability and guide evaluation.

CHAPTER 82

VENA CAVAL FILTERS: THE PREPIC TRIAL

Anish Mehta

A Clinical Trial of Vena Caval Filters in the Prevention of Pulmonary Embolism in Patients With Proximal Deep-Vein Thrombosis

Decousus H, Leizorovicz A, Parent F, et al. *N Engl J Med.* 1998;338(7):409–415

BACKGROUND

The primary indication for vena caval (VC) filter placement is for patients with deep venous thrombosis (DVT) who cannot receive anticoagulant therapy. As VC filters became safer to place in the years preceding this study, they were often used in conjunction with anticoagulation based on observational studies suggesting additional benefit in reducing the incidence of pulmonary embolism (PE). However, no high-quality evidence existed to guide this practice.

OBJECTIVES

To determine whether VC filters are effective at preventing PE in high-risk patients with DVT. (The trial also compared the efficacy of low–molecular-weight heparin versus unfractionated heparin, an objective not covered in this chapter.)

METHODS

Randomized, open-label trial at 44 French centers between 1991 and 1995. The trial used a 2-by-2 factorial design to investigate both VC filter placement and anticoagulant choice, only the former of which is reported below.

Patients

400 adult patients. Inclusion criteria included hospitalization with acute proximal DVT confirmed by venography (with or without concomitant pulmonary embolus) and high risk for PE (determined by physician assessment). Exclusion criteria included placement of previous filter, contraindication to or failure of anticoagulant therapy, anticoagulant therapy lasting >48 hours by the time of randomization, indication for thrombolysis, and short life expectancy.

Interventions

VC filter versus no filter, and unfractionated versus low–molecular-weight heparin. (This chapter focuses exclusively on the filter comparisons.) Patients were bridged to oral (when possible) or subcutaneous anticoagulant therapy for ≥3 months.

Outcomes

The primary outcome was the occurrence of new PE (symptomatic or asymptomatic) within 12 days after randomization. Secondary outcomes included death and any symptomatic events (including PE, recurrent DVT, filter complications, and major bleeding) within 2 years after randomization.

KEY RESULTS
- By day 12, the VC filter group had a lower rate of new PE (1.1% vs. 4.8%, OR = 0.22, 95% CI 0.05–0.90, $p = 0.03$).
- By 2 years, both groups had similar rates of symptomatic PE (3.4% vs. 6.3%, OR = 0.50, 95% CI 0.19–1.33, $p = 0.16$) and death (21.6% vs. 20.1%, OR = 1.10, 95% CI 0.72–1.70, $p = 0.65$).
- By 2 years, the VC filter group had a higher rate of recurrent DVT (20.8% vs. 11.6%, OR = 1.87, 95% CI 1.10–3.20, $p = 0.02$).

STUDY CONCLUSIONS
The short-term benefit of VC filters in preventing new PE was outweighed by a lack of mortality benefit and increased risk of recurrent DVT after 2 years.

COMMENTARY

The PREPIC results substantially changed the indications for placement of VC filters, and an 8-year follow-up of this cohort confirmed the increased risk of DVT and lack of long-term mortality benefit. Retrievable VC filters, which were subsequently developed and are theoretically safer, have led to continued variability in the use of these devices; these are currently being evaluated in ongoing randomized studies. The 2016 American College of Chest Physicians guidelines recommend against VC filters in patients with acute DVT or PE who are treated with anticoagulants.

Question
Should high-risk patients with acute DVT who can tolerate anticoagulation receive a VC filter to prevent PE?

Answer
No, VC filters offer no benefit in morbidity and mortality over anticoagulation alone, and may cause harm.

CHAPTER 83

THROMBOLYSIS IN ACUTE PULMONARY EMBOLISM

Viswatej Avutu

Alteplase Versus Heparin in Acute Pulmonary Embolism: Randomised Trial Assessing Right-Ventricular Function and Pulmonary Perfusion

Goldhaber SZ, Haire WD, Feldstein ML, et al. *Lancet.* 1993;341(8844):507–511

BACKGROUND

Prior studies had suggested that thrombolysis with recombinant tissue-type plasminogen activator (rt-PA) followed by anticoagulation could improve right ventricular (RV) dysfunction and pulmonary perfusion in patients with acute pulmonary embolism (PE). However, prospective randomized data of this association were lacking.

OBJECTIVES

To determine whether rt-PA followed by heparin was superior to heparin alone in acute PE for improving RV function and pulmonary perfusion and reducing adverse clinical outcomes.

METHODS

Randomized, double-blind trial at 9 US hospitals between 1988 and 1991.

Patients

101 patients. Inclusion criteria included age ≥18 years with confirmed PE, either by high probability ventilation–perfusion lung scans and/or pulmonary angiograms. Exclusion criteria included major internal bleeding within previous 6 months, intracranial or intraspinal disease, severe hepatic dysfunction, pregnancy, infective endocarditis, or expected survival ≤1 month.

Interventions

Intravenous rt-PA (100 mg over 2 hours) followed by intravenous heparin (continuous infusion with goal PTT 1.5×–2.5× upper limit of normal) versus intravenous heparin alone (bolus followed by continuous infusion). All patients were subsequently bridged to oral anticoagulation.

Outcomes

The primary outcome was RV function (as assessed by RV wall motion and end-diastolic area via echocardiogram). Secondary outcomes included pulmonary tissue perfusion as assessed by lung perfusion scan and incidence of clinically suspected recurrent PE. Adverse events included death and clinically suspected recurrent PE within 14 days and bleeding (intracranial bleeding, bleeding that required surgery, >0.1 drop in hematocrit) within 72 hours.

KEY RESULTS

- Patients receiving rt-PA had higher rates of improvement (39% vs. 17%) and lower rates of worsening (2% vs. 17%) in RV wall motion by 24 hours ($p = 0.005$) compared to baseline, a finding that was even more pronounced for patients with baseline RV hypokinesis.
- Patients receiving rt-PA had higher rates of improvement in pulmonary perfusion (14.6% vs. 1.5%, $p < 0.0001$).
- There was no statistically significant difference in the number of patients experiencing recurrent PE within 14 days (0 among those receiving rt-PA and heparin vs. 5 among those receiving heparin alone, $p = 0.06$).
- Bleeding with >0.1 drop in hematocrit was rare (1 in each group; only patient in rt-PA group requiring transfusion).

STUDY CONCLUSIONS

When used with heparin, rt-PA rapidly improves RV function and pulmonary perfusion among patients with PE.

COMMENTARY

This trial solidified the idea that thrombolysis can improve RV function and pulmonary perfusion in acute PE compared to anticoagulation alone. These results, along with those from complementary studies, have helped establish thrombolysis as one possible management option for patients with acute PE and RV dysfunction. However, caveats include small sample size and lack of meaningful endpoints (death, bleeding complications) beyond 14 days. Moreover, subsequent evaluations have revealed the significant bleeding risks associated with thrombolysis while also failing to demonstrate benefit in those with stable PE. In turn, guidelines now recommend rt-PA largely for patients with hemodynamically unstable PE.[1,2]

Question

Should thrombolysis, in addition to heparin therapy, be considered in patients with hemodynamically unstable PE?

Answer

Yes, although other factors, including bleeding risk and response to resuscitation, should also be considered.

References

1. Konstantinides SV, Torbicki A, Agnelli G, et al; Task Force for the Diagnosis and Management of Acute Pulmonary Embolism of the European Society of Cardiology (ESC). 2014 ESC guidelines on the diagnosis and management of acute pulmonary embolism. *Eur Heart J.* 2014;35(43):3033–3069.
2. Kearon C, Akl EA, Ornelas J, et al. Antithrombotic therapy for VTE disease: CHEST Guideline and Expert Panel Report. *Chest.* 2016;149(2):315–352.

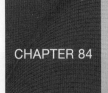

COMBINATION LONG-ACTING BETA AGONIST AND INHALED CORTICOSTEROID IN COPD: THE TORCH TRIAL

Amy O. Flaster

Salmeterol and Fluticasone Propionate and Survival in Chronic Obstructive Pulmonary Disease

Calverley PM, Anderson JA, Celli B, et al. *N Engl J Med.* 2007;356(8):775–789

BACKGROUND

At the time of this study, no pharmacologic therapy had demonstrated a direct effect on mortality in patients with chronic obstructive pulmonary disease (COPD). The only existing data consisted of retrospective studies that suggested a mortality benefit from inhaled corticosteroids and combination corticosteroids with long-acting beta agonists.

OBJECTIVES

To determine the effect of combined long-acting beta agonist and inhaled corticosteroid therapy on COPD mortality.

METHODS

Randomized, double-blind, placebo-controlled trial at 444 centers in 42 countries on 5 continents.

Patients

6,112 patients with COPD confirmed by spirometry. Inclusion criteria included age 40 to 80 years, ≥ 10 pack-year smoking history, and FEV_1 <60% predicted. Exclusion criteria included long-term home oxygen therapy, current oral corticosteroid use, or concurrent non-COPD respiratory disorder.

Interventions

There were 4 treatment arms: combination therapy (salmeterol and fluticasone) versus salmeterol versus fluticasone versus placebo. All drugs were taken twice daily for 3 years.

Outcomes

The primary outcome was time to death from any cause by 3 years. Secondary outcomes included frequency of COPD exacerbations, lung function (by spirometry), and health status (by a validated, disease-specific questionnaire).

KEY RESULTS

- At 3 years, mortality was 12.6% in the combination therapy group, 13.5% in the salmeterol group, 16.0% in the fluticasone group, and 15.2% in the placebo group. The HR for death in the combination therapy group compared to placebo was 0.825 (95% CI 0.681–1.002, $p = 0.052$).
- The rate of COPD exacerbation was lower in the combination group than in the placebo group (0.85/year vs. 1.13/year, RR 0.75, 95% CI 0.69–0.81, $p < 0.001$).
- Annual rates of hospital admission for COPD exacerbation were lower in the combination and salmeterol groups than in the placebo group ($p = 0.03$ and $p = 0.02$, respectively).
- The probability of having pneumonia in the combination, salmeterol, fluticasone, and placebo groups was 19.6%, 13.3%, 18.3%, and 12.3%, respectively. These probabilities were statistically significantly higher in the combination and fluticasone groups compared to placebo ($p < 0.001$ for both comparisons).

STUDY CONCLUSIONS

Treatment with combination salmeterol-fluticasone propionate did not reduce mortality compared with placebo, but did result in fewer COPD exacerbations.

COMMENTARY

Though it did not demonstrate a statistically significant mortality reduction, TORCH reported impressive effects on other clinically relevant endpoints. Through post hoc factorial analysis, some argued that the benefits of combination therapy were entirely attributable to salmeterol. Others claimed that the addition of inhaled corticosteroids was actually harmful, pointing to other research that confirmed the higher risk of pneumonia in steroid-containing treatment arms. Despite these criticisms, TORCH's large size and long duration of follow-up are noteworthy, and the study has had a significant impact on modern COPD management. The 2016 Global Initiative for Chronic Obstructive Lung Disease guidelines recommend combination long-acting beta agonist and inhaled corticosteroid therapy for high-risk patients with or without severe symptoms.

Question

Should patients with moderate-to-severe COPD receive combination long-acting beta agonist and inhaled corticosteroid therapy?

Answer

Yes, although combination therapy has not been definitively shown to provide a survival benefit, it reduces the frequency and severity of COPD exacerbations.

CHAPTER 85

DABIGATRAN FOR THE TREATMENT OF VENOUS THROMBOEMBOLISM: THE RE-COVER TRIAL

Anthony Carnicelli

Dabigatran Versus Warfarin in the Treatment of Acute Venous Thromboembolism

Schulman S, Kearon C, Kakkar AK, et al. *N Engl J Med.* 2009;361(24):2342–2352

BACKGROUND

Prior to this study, warfarin had long been the gold standard and only oral anticoagulant approved for the treatment of acute venous thromboembolism (VTE). However, warfarin interacts with many foods and drugs and requires frequent blood testing and dose adjustment. In contrast, dabigatran is a direct thrombin inhibitor that does not require coagulation monitoring and possesses a fixed dosing schedule, rapid onset of action, predictable anticoagulant effect, and fewer potential food and drug interactions.

OBJECTIVES

To compare the safety and efficacy of dabigatran versus warfarin for the treatment of acute VTE.

METHODS

Randomized, double-blind, double-dummy, noninferiority trial at 228 sites in 29 countries between 2006 and 2008. Sham INR testing was utilized in the dabigatran group to maintain blinding.

Patients

2,564 patients. Inclusion criteria included acute symptomatic proximal deep vein thrombosis of the legs or pulmonary embolism diagnosed by imaging. Exclusion criteria included symptoms >14 days, hemodynamic instability, thrombolysis, high bleeding risk, and other indications for warfarin.

Interventions

Dabigatran (150 mg twice daily) versus warfarin (goal INR 2.0 to 3.0).

Outcomes

The primary outcome was 6-month incidence of recurrent symptomatic VTE or related deaths. Safety outcomes included bleeding (major, clinically relevant nonmajor, and any) events.

KEY RESULTS

- Dabigatran was noninferior to warfarin with respect to 6-month incidence of recurrent symptomatic VTE or related deaths (HR 1.10, 95% CI 0.65–1.84, $p < 0.001$ for noninferiority).
- Dabigatran was associated with lower rates of major or clinically relevant nonmajor bleeding (HR 0.63, 95% CI 0.47–0.84, $p = 0.002$) and any bleeding (HR 0.71, 95% CI 0.59–0.85, $p < 0.001$); the 2 groups had similar rates of major bleeding (HR 0.82, 95% CI 0.45–1.48, $p = 0.38$).
- There were no statistically significant differences in frequency of adverse events except for dyspepsia, which occurred more frequently in the dabigatran group (2.9% vs. 0.6%, $p < 0.001$).

STUDY CONCLUSIONS

For the treatment of acute VTE, dabigatran is as effective as warfarin and has a similar safety profile.

COMMENTARY

As the first trial to show the efficacy and safety of an oral anticoagulant compared to warfarin, RE-COVER began the shift toward the use of direct oral anticoagulants (DOACs) in acute VTE. Its findings are particularly notable given that dabigatran was noninferior compared to a warfarin group with a higher average time in therapeutic INR range (60%) than has been estimated in real world settings. The study's main conclusion – that DOACs are comparable in efficacy and safety to warfarin – has been reinforced in studies of other agents such as rivaroxaban (EINSTEIN[1]), apixaban (AMPLIFY[2]), and edoxaban (Hokusai-VTE[3]). Collectively, these studies have produced changes in the 2016 American College of Chest Physicians VTE guidelines, which recommend DOACs over warfarin for the treatment of VTE in patients without malignancy.

Question

Can DOACs be used for the treatment of acute symptomatic VTE?

Answer

Yes, a number of agents can be used effectively and safely for this indication.

References

1. Bauersachs R, Berkowitz SD, Brenner B, et al; EINSTEIN Investigators. Oral rivaroxaban for symptomatic venous thromboembolism. *N Engl J Med.* 2010;363(26):2499–2510.
2. Agnelli G, Buller HR, Cohen A, et al; AMPLIFY Investigators. Oral apixaban for the treatment of acute venous thromboembolism. *N Engl J Med.* 2013;369(9):799–808.
3. Büller HR, Décousus H, Grosso MA, et al; Hokusai-VTE Investigators. Edoxaban versus warfarin for the treatment of symptomatic venous thromboembolism. *N Engl J Med.* 2013;369(15):1406–1415.

CHAPTER 86

NONINVASIVE VENTILATION FOR COPD EXACERBATIONS

Elizabeth A. Richey

Noninvasive Ventilation for Acute Exacerbations of Chronic Obstructive Pulmonary Disease

Brochard L, Mancebo J, Wysocki M, et al. *N Engl J Med.* 1995;333(13):817–822

BACKGROUND

By reducing the need for intubation and risk of associated complications, noninvasive ventilation represents an alternative for treating the often rapidly reversible respiratory failure caused by acute exacerbations of chronic obstructive pulmonary disease (COPD). Prior to this study, however, the vast majority of evidence supporting noninvasive ventilation in these situations had come from observational studies. Prospective data on its effects on morbidity, mortality, and in-hospital events were lacking.

OBJECTIVE

To evaluate the efficacy of noninvasive ventilation compared to standard medical treatment for acute exacerbations of COPD.

METHODS

Randomized, unblinded trial at 5 sites in 3 European countries between 1990 and 1991.

Patients

85 patients with acute COPD exacerbations. Inclusion criteria included known COPD (defined by known diagnosis or compatible history, physical examination, and chest radiograph), respiratory acidosis, an elevated bicarbonate level, and ≥ 2 of the following after 10 minutes breathing room air: respiratory rate >30, PaO_2 <45 mm Hg, and pH <7.35. Exclusion criteria included refusal to undergo intubation, respiratory rate <12, or the need for immediate intubation at time of screening (e.g., recent receipt of sedative medications, primary central nervous system or neuromuscular disorder, cardiac arrest within 5 days, cardiogenic pulmonary edema, upper airway obstruction or asthma, and specific causes of decompensation such as peritonitis or pneumothorax requiring specific treatment).

Interventions

Noninvasive positive pressure ventilation (via face mask for ≥ 6 hr/day on standardized equipment) versus standard treatment (supplemental oxygen via nasal cannula at a maximal flow rate of 5 L/min and target oxygen saturation >90%).

Outcomes

The primary outcome was the need for endotracheal intubation and mechanical ventilation at any time during hospitalization. Secondary outcomes included length of hospital stay, complications of hospitalization, duration of ventilator assistance, and in-hospital mortality.

KEY RESULTS

- Patients receiving noninvasive ventilation had lower rates of endotracheal intubation (26% vs. 74%, $p < 0.001$), rates of complications (16% vs. 48%, $p = 0.001$), and shorter hospital stays (23 ± 17 days vs. 35 ± 33 days, $p = 0.005$).
- Patients receiving noninvasive ventilation had lower in-hospital mortality (9% vs. 29%, $p = 0.02$), with no statistically significant difference between the 2 groups after adjustment for endotracheal intubation rates.

STUDY CONCLUSIONS

In selected patients with acute COPD exacerbations, noninvasive ventilation can reduce the need for endotracheal intubation, the length of the hospital stay, and the in-hospital mortality rate.

COMMENTARY

By providing definitive evidence for noninvasive ventilation in acute COPD exacerbations, this trial encouraged investments in training and resources for routine use of this therapy. Of note, certain respiratory treatments – including oxygenation face mask or high flow nasal cannula oxygen delivery – were not available as part of the standard treatment arm in this trial, and not all patients received anticholinergic agents. Along with subsequent work, the findings of this study contributed to the 2016 Global Initiative for Chronic Obstructive Lung Disease guidelines, which note that in all but a few situations, it is reasonable to trial noninvasive ventilation among patients with acute COPD exacerbations in an effort to minimize invasive mechanical ventilation and its complications.

Question

In patients with acute exacerbations of COPD, is it appropriate to trial noninvasive ventilation as a first treatment option?

Answer

Yes, noninvasive ventilation helps reduce endotracheal intubation, complications, and length of hospital stay.

CHAPTER 87

LMWH FOR VTE PROPHYLAXIS: THE MEDENOX TRIAL

Amy O. Flaster

A Comparison of Enoxaparin With Placebo for the Prevention of Venous Thromboembolism in Acutely Ill Medical Patients

Samama MM, Cohen AT, Darmon JY, et al. *N Engl J Med.* 1999;341(11):793–800

BACKGROUND

At the time of this study, data strongly supported routine thromboprophylaxis in surgical inpatients. However, the practice was controversial in general medical inpatients. Outside of those with stroke or myocardial infarction, the burden of VTE in such patients was unknown, and studies assessing the benefit of prophylactic anticoagulation on medical wards assessed very heterogeneous populations and had inconsistent results.

OBJECTIVES

To determine the frequency of venous thromboembolism in medical inpatients and assess the safety and efficacy of low–molecular-weight heparin (LMWH) regimens for thromboprophylaxis.

METHODS

Randomized, double-blind, placebo-controlled trial at 60 centers in 9 countries in Europe, North America, and the Middle East between 1996 and 1998.

Patients

1,102 patients who were projected to be in the hospital for ≥6 days without being immobilized for >3 days. Inclusion criteria included age >40 years, a common medical admitting diagnosis, and ≥1 additional VTE risk factor. Exclusion criteria included pregnancy, thrombophilia, recent stroke or major surgery, uncontrolled hypertension, active peptic ulcer disease, intubation, or serum creatinine >1.7 mg/dL.

Interventions

Enoxaparin 40 mg daily versus enoxaparin 20 mg daily versus placebo for 6 to 14 days while in the hospital.

Outcomes

The primary outcome was the development of VTE, defined as deep venous thrombosis (DVT), pulmonary embolism (PE), or both, between days 1 and 14. All patients were assessed with lower extremity contrast venography or ultrasonography between days 6 and 14, or earlier if symptomatic. Suspected PE was confirmed by lung scan, angiography, computed tomography, or autopsy. Secondary outcomes included hemorrhage and death.

KEY RESULTS

- VTE prevalence by day 14 was lower in the enoxaparin 40 mg group than in the placebo group (5.5% vs. 14.9%, RR 0.37, 95% CI 0.22–0.63, $p < 0.001$). There was no difference between the 20 mg and placebo groups ($p = 0.90$).
- By day 14, PE rates were low across treatment arms, ranging from 0% in the enoxaparin 40 mg group to 1.0% in the placebo group.
- Rates of major hemorrhage were 1.7%, 0.3%, and 1.1% in the enoxaparin 40 mg, 20 mg, and placebo groups, respectively. Risk of death from any cause was low and did not vary between enoxaparin and placebo groups (RR = 0.83, 95% CI 0.56–1.21, $p = 0.31$ for 40 mg and 1.05, 95% CI 0.71–1.56, $p = 0.80$ for 20 mg).

STUDY CONCLUSIONS

Enoxaparin 40 mg daily prevented VTE in medical inpatients without significantly increasing the risk of major bleeding.

COMMENTARY

MEDENOX was the first of 3 major clinical trials (the others being PREVENT,[1] which assessed dalteparin, and ARTEMIS,[2] which tested fondaparinux) to establish gold standards for thromboprophylaxis in medical inpatients. These studies clarified the benefits of what had previously been inconsistent clinical practice. MEDENOX was criticized because 22% of patients were not included in the primary analysis, most often because their venograms were not evaluable, though the proportion of nonincluded patients were roughly equal across treatment arms. As a result of this triad of studies, the 2008 American College of Chest Physicians VTE prophylaxis guidelines recommend LMWH as a first-line option for medical inpatients with characteristics similar to those in the trials.

Question

Should thromboprophylaxis be used in hospitalized general medical patients at elevated risk for VTE?

Answer

Yes, thromboprophylaxis prevents VTE in high-risk medical inpatients.

References

1. Leizorovicz A, Cohen AT, Turpie AG, et al. Randomized, placebo-controlled trial of dalteparin for the prevention of venous thromboembolism in acutely ill medical patients. *Circulation*. 2004;110(7):874–879.
2. Cohen AT, Davidson BL, Gallus AS, et al. Efficacy and safety of fondaparinux for the prevention of venous thromboembolism in older acute medical patients: randomised placebo controlled trial. *BMJ*. 2006;332(7537):325–329.

CHAPTER 88

LIGHT'S CRITERIA FOR PLEURAL EFFUSIONS

Elizabeth A. Richey

Pleural Effusions: The Diagnostic Separation of Transudates and Exudates

Light RW, MacGregor MI, Luchsinger PC, Ball WC Jr., *Ann Intern Med.* 1972;77(4): 507–513

BACKGROUND

Pleural effusions are typically categorized as transudates or exudates, with transudates suggesting systemic conditions (e.g., heart failure and cirrhosis) and exudates signaling inflammation with pleural involvement (e.g., from malignancy, pneumonia, and tuberculosis). Prior to this study, the use of pleural fluid total protein level led to frequent misclassification of transudates and exudates. Pleural lactic dehydrogenase (LDH) had been proposed as an alternative, but the utility of using LDH and other laboratory values to classify pleural effusions was unknown.

OBJECTIVES

To determine the utility of pleural fluid cell count, protein levels, and LDH levels for differentiating between transudates and exudates.

METHODS

Descriptive study at 2 US hospitals between 1970 and 1971.

Patients

150 patients from medical wards at The Johns Hopkins Hospital and The Good Samaritan Hospital who presented with pleural effusions and underwent thoracentesis.

Intervention

Patients were diagnosed and classified based on predefined clinical criteria with conditions that cause transudates (heart failure, cirrhosis, and nephrosis) or exudates (malignancy, pneumonia, tuberculosis, and other inflammatory conditions). Serum and pleural samples were obtained to measure serum protein and LDH, and pleural LDH, protein, and cell counts. Values were plotted graphically by clinical diagnosis. 33 effusions corresponding to patients who could not be classified were excluded.

Outcomes

Characteristics, determined by graphical plots of laboratory values as functions of patient diagnoses, for distinguishing between transudates and exudates:

- A pleural fluid:serum protein ratio >0.5
- A pleural fluid:serum LDH ratio >0.6
- A pleural fluid LDH >200 IU (with upper limit of normal of 300 IU)

KEY RESULTS

- Each of the 3 characteristics correctly identified >70% of the exudates and at most 1 of the transudates.
- 99% of the exudative effusions met at least 1 of the 3 characteristics.
- Cell count was of limited use for separating transudates from exudates.
- Most exudative effusions, not only malignant effusions, had high pleural fluid LDH level.

STUDY CONCLUSIONS

The presence of any 1 of the following 3 characteristics – a pleural fluid-to-serum protein ratio >0.5, a pleural fluid-to-serum LDH ratio >0.6, or a pleural fluid LDH >200 IU – indicates that a pleural effusion is an exudate.

COMMENTARY

These 3 characteristics (which came to be known as "Light's criteria") continue to be relevant today as a common first screen for identifying exudative effusions. Several design choices – reliance on clinical criteria as the gold standard, exclusion of cases that could not be classified, and selection of criteria that provided high sensitivity for identifying exudates – may help contextualize subsequent studies showing that 15% to 20% of transudates can be misclassified by these criteria. In cases with high pretest probability of transudative fluid, Light's criteria can be considered alongside serum-pleural fluid protein gradient or serum-pleural fluid albumin gradient to improve classification.

Question

Are Light's criteria an effective tool for identifying exudative pleural effusions?

Answer

Yes, nearly all exudates are appropriately identified, but other measures should be considered to avoid misclassification of transudates.

CHAPTER 89

LONG-ACTING MUSCARINIC THERAPY IN COPD

Ersilia M. DeFilippis

Prevention of Exacerbations of Chronic Obstructive Pulmonary Disease with Tiotropium, a Once-Daily Inhaled Anticholinergic Bronchodilator: A Randomized Trial

Niewoehner DE, Rice K, Cote C, et al. *Ann Int Med.* 2005;143(5):317–326

BACKGROUND

At the time of this study, relatively few agents had been shown to prevent exacerbations of chronic obstructive pulmonary disease (COPD). Prior studies had shown improvements in health-related quality of life and lung function with tiotropium, but its impact on other clinical outcomes was unproven.

OBJECTIVES

To evaluate the efficacy of tiotropium in reducing COPD exacerbations and hospitalizations.

METHODS

Randomized, double-blind, placebo-controlled trial in 26 American centers from 2001 to 2003.

Patients

1,829 patients. Inclusion criteria included moderate to severe COPD (FEV_1 ≤60% predicted and FEV_1/FVC ≤70% predicted), age ≥40 years, and ≥10 pack-year smoking history. Exclusion criteria included serious arrhythmia, myocardial infarction within 6 months, heart failure admission in the last year, asthma, or recent unresolved COPD exacerbation.

Intervention

Tiotropium (18 µg inhaled daily) or placebo. All patients continued their usual medications but were not permitted to take any open-label short- or long-acting anticholinergics.

Outcomes

Coprimary outcomes were percentage of patients with ≥1 COPD exacerbation and percentage with ≥1 COPD exacerbation hospitalization during the treatment period (6 months). Secondary outcomes included time to first exacerbation, spirometry, days of antibiotic treatment for COPD, and days of systemic corticosteroid therapy for COPD.

KEY RESULTS

- Treatment with tiotropium was associated with fewer COPD exacerbations (27.9% vs. 32.3%, $p = 0.037$).
- There were no statistically significant differences between the 2 groups in frequency of hospitalization for COPD exacerbation (7.0% vs. 9.5%, $p = 0.056$).
- FEV_1 response was improved in the tiotropium group at 90 and 180 days ($p < 0.001$).
- Tiotropium reduced unscheduled medical visits for COPD exacerbation ($p = 0.019$) and days of antibiotic therapy ($p = 0.015$).

STUDY CONCLUSIONS

Treatment with tiotropium reduces COPD exacerbations in patients with moderate to severe COPD.

COMMENTARY

This large, multicenter trial demonstrated modest, but clinically relevant, improvements in key outcomes with a new class of medication. Limitations include short follow-up time and use of placebo control, with participants taken off their home ipratropium inhalers rather than allowing direct comparison between tiotropium and ipratropium. The authors later demonstrated that the placebo group did not experience adverse effects from cessation of their prestudy inhaler therapy. Tiotropium's benefit has since been confirmed in more heterogeneous populations and with significantly longer follow-up times. However, there is conflicting evidence regarding tiotropium's cardiovascular safety,[1,2] a finding accentuated by the fact that many cardiac patients were excluded from this trial. The 2016 Global Initiative for Chronic Obstructive Lung Disease COPD management guidelines recommend long-acting anticholinergic agents as first-line options for symptomatic and/or high-risk patients.

Question

Is tiotropium a reasonable option for patients with moderate to severe COPD?

Answer

Yes, tiotropium reduces the risk of COPD exacerbations in patients with moderate-to-severe disease.

References

1. Singh S, Loke YK, Furberg CD. Inhaled anticholinergics and risk of major adverse cardiovascular events in patients with chronic obstructive pulmonary disease: a systematic review and meta-analysis. *JAMA.* 2008;300(12):1439–1450.
2. Celli B, Decramer M, Leimer I, Vogel U, Kesten S, Tashkin DP. Cardiovascular safety of tiotropium in patients with COPD. *Chest.* 2010;137(1):20–30.

CHAPTER 90

INHALED CORTICOSTEROIDS IN COPD

Kristin Castillo Farias

Multicentre Randomized Placebo-Controlled Trial of Inhaled Fluticasone Propionate in Patients With Chronic Obstructive Pulmonary Disease

Paggiaro PL, Dahle R, Bakran I, et al. *Lancet.* 1998;351(9105):773–780

BACKGROUND

By the late 1990s, inhaled corticosteroid (ICS) therapy had been shown to prevent exacerbations and improve pulmonary function and quality of life in patients with asthma. However, the clinical effects of ICS monotherapy in COPD were not as clear, leading to inconsistent uptake of ICS therapy in clinical practice.

OBJECTIVES

To investigate the efficacy of fluticasone propionate in patients with COPD.

METHODS

Randomized, double-blind, placebo-controlled trial across 13 European countries, New Zealand, and South Africa between 1993 and 1995.

Patients

281 patients. Inclusion criteria included age 50 to 75 years, persistent symptoms (via daily record cards) after withholding baseline ICS medications during a 2-week washout period, chronic bronchitis (productive cough $\geq$3 months for $\geq$2 years without other cause), $\geq$10 pack-year smoking history, predicted FEV_1 35% to 90%, FEV_1/FVC $\leq$70%, lack of bronchodilator reversibility, and $\geq$1 exacerbation per year for the previous 3 years. Exclusion criteria included abnormal chest x-ray, use of systemic steroids, receipt of antibiotic therapy, use of ICS >500 µg daily or inhaled fluticasone, or hospitalization in the prior 4 weeks.

Interventions

Fluticasone propionate (500 mg inhaled twice daily) versus placebo.

Outcomes

The primary outcome was the number of patients with $\geq$1 exacerbation at 6 months. Exacerbations were defined as worsening of symptoms requiring change in treatment and were categorized as "mild" (self-managed at home), "moderate" (outpatient treatment by a physician), and "severe" (hospitalization). Secondary outcomes included number and severity of exacerbations, lung function, symptoms, peak expiratory flow, and 6-minute walk distance.

KEY RESULTS

- There was no difference in the number of patients with ≥1 exacerbation (32% in the fluticasone group vs. 37% in the placebo group, $p = 0.449$).
- Fewer patients in the fluticasone group had moderate or severe exacerbations (60% vs. 86%, $p < 0.001$).
- Compared to those taking placebo, the fluticasone group had improved peak expiratory flows ($p = 0.048$) and FEV_1 ($p < 0.001$).
- The fluticasone group had lower symptom scores for median daily cough ($p = 0.004$) and sputum volume ($p = 0.016$) without statistically significant effects on breathlessness or need for bronchodilators.
- Fluticasone was associated with a greater increase in adjusted 6-minute walk distance (27 m vs. 8 m, $p = 0.032$).

STUDY CONCLUSIONS

Treatment of COPD patients with fluticasone resulted in a reduction of moderate to severe exacerbations, improvement of symptoms, and improvements in 6-minute walk distance.

COMMENTARY

This was the first trial to study the effects of high-dose ICS monotherapy against placebo in patients diagnosed with COPD using spirometry, a uniquely stringent diagnostic standard at the time which allowed asthma patients to be excluded. Subsequent evaluations have confirmed many of this study's findings while also demonstrating an increased risk of pneumonia with prolonged ICS use. Though later research shifted practice away from lone ICS in COPD, the 2016 Global Initiative for Chronic Obstructive Lung Disease guidelines continue to recommend the addition of ICS therapy to long-acting bronchodilators in patients at high risk of exacerbations.

Question

Is it reasonable to treat patients who are at high risk of COPD exacerbation with an ICS?

Answer

Yes, despite the risk of pneumonia, ICS therapy reduces exacerbations and improves symptoms and should be used in combination with a long-acting beta agonist.

CHAPTER 91

GLUCOCORTICOIDS FOR COPD EXACERBATIONS

Elizabeth A. Richey

Effect of Systemic Glucocorticoids on Exacerbations of Chronic Obstructive Pulmonary Disease

Niewoehner DE, Erbland ML, Deupree RH, et al. *N Engl J Med.* 1999;340(25): 1941–1947

BACKGROUND

Although systemic glucocorticoids were standard treatment for patients hospitalized with COPD exacerbations leading up to this study, prospective data about their efficacy and effect on clinical outcomes were lacking. Despite the potential for systemic glucocorticoids to cause short- and long-term complications, the optimal treatment duration also remained unknown.

OBJECTIVES

To evaluate the efficacy of systemic glucocorticoids in the treatment of COPD exacerbations.

METHODS

Randomized, double-blind trial at 25 US centers between 1994 and 1996.

Patients

271 patients. Inclusion criteria included clinical diagnosis of COPD exacerbation, age ≥50 years, ≥30 pack-year smoking history, and FEV1 <1.5 L or inability to perform spirometry due to dyspnea. Exclusion criteria included treatment with glucocorticoids within the last month.

Interventions

Systemic glucocorticoids (8 weeks) versus systemic glucocorticoids followed by placebo (2 weeks of glucocorticoids, 6 weeks of placebo) versus placebo (8 weeks). Patients in the 2 glucocorticoid groups received 125 mg of intravenous methylprednisolone every 6 hours for the first 72 hours, followed by a tapered course of daily oral prednisone starting with 60 mg daily.

Outcomes

The primary outcome was treatment failure, defined as a composite of death from any cause, need for intubation and mechanical ventilation, readmission to the hospital for COPD, or intensification of drug therapy. Secondary outcomes included length of hospital stay, death from any cause within a 6-month follow-up period, and complications including hyperglycemia, hypertension, and secondary infections.

KEY RESULTS

- Compared to placebo, patients receiving glucocorticoids had lower rates of treatment failure at 30 days (23% vs. 33%, $p = 0.04$) and 90 days (37% vs. 48%, $p = 0.04$), as well as shorter initial hospital stays (8.5 days vs. 9.7 days, $p = 0.03$).
- The duration of glucocorticoid therapy (8 weeks vs. 2 weeks) had no significant effect on the primary outcome of treatment failure at 30 or 90 days.
- Patients receiving glucocorticoids experienced hyperglycemia requiring treatment more frequently (15% vs. 4%, $p = 0.002$), but there were no statistically significant differences in the time spent in the hospital for reasons other than COPD (4.4 days vs. 1.2 days, $p = 0.07$).

STUDY CONCLUSIONS

Among patients hospitalized with COPD exacerbations, treatment with systemic glucocorticoids results in moderate improvement in clinical outcomes, with maximal benefit during the first 2 weeks of therapy.

COMMENTARY

This trial was pivotal in establishing both the effect of systemic glucocorticoids on clinical outcomes in the treatment of COPD exacerbation and the lack of utility in treating for >2 weeks. The doses administered in the trial could have led to the high rate of observed complications and increased hospital stays, and subsequent work has demonstrated the efficacy of lower doses and shorter treatment duration. Based on this collective evidence, the 2016 Global Initiative for Chronic Obstructive Lung Disease guidelines recommend short courses of systemic glucocorticoids, preferably via the oral route and for as short as 5 days to minimize complications, for treatment of COPD exacerbation.

Question

Should patients experiencing COPD exacerbations receive systemic glucocorticoids?

Answer

Yes, although the dose and duration, as well as patient-specific factors (e.g., history of hyperglycemia), must be considered to balance the adverse and beneficial effects of treatment.

| CHAPTER 92 | DUAL THERAPY IN ASTHMA: THE FACET STUDY |

Neelam A. Phadke

Effect of Inhaled Formoterol and Budesonide on Exacerbations of Asthma.
Pauwels RA, Löfdahl CG, Postma DS, et al. *N Engl J Med.* 1997;337(20):1405–1411

BACKGROUND

Despite first-line inhaled corticosteroid (ICS) treatment, patients with moderate to severe, persistent asthma frequently need additional treatment, such as inhaled β_2-agonists, for symptom control. At the time of this study, there was inconclusive evidence regarding the efficacy of long-acting β_2-agonists (LABAs) with small reports suggesting an increased rate of hospitalizations and more severe exacerbations with these medications.

OBJECTIVES

To determine the effect of adding the inhaled LABA formoterol to the ICS budesonide on asthma outcomes.

METHODS

Randomized, double-blind trial at 71 centers in 9 countries on 3 continents from 1994 to 1995.

Patients

694 patients. Inclusion criteria included age 18 to 70 years, asthma for ≥6 months treated with an ICS for ≥3 months, and baseline FEV_1 ≥50% predicted value with ≥15% increase with terbutaline. Exclusion criteria included treatment with high-dose ICS, frequent use of oral glucocorticoids, or asthma hospitalization in the previous 6 months.

Interventions

There were 4 treatment groups: low-dose budesonide (100 µg twice daily) plus placebo versus low-dose budesonide plus formoterol (12 µg twice daily) versus high-dose budesonide (400 µg twice daily) plus placebo versus high-dose budesonide plus formoterol. All patients received 800 µg inhaled budesonide twice daily and 250 µg terbutaline as needed for 4 weeks before randomization.

Outcomes

The 2 primary outcomes were rates of mild and severe asthma exacerbations per patient per year. Secondary outcomes included symptom scores and asthma hospitalizations. The study was analyzed in a 2-by-2 factorial manner.

KEY RESULTS

- Compared to placebo, formoterol was associated with a lower rate of mild ($p < 0.001$) and severe ($p = 0.01$) exacerbations, as well as lower nighttime ($p < 0.001$) and daytime ($p < 0.001$) symptom scores.
- Compared to low-dose budesonide, high-dose budesonide was associated with a lower rate of mild ($p < 0.001$) and severe ($p < 0.001$) exacerbations, as well as lower daytime symptom scores ($p = 0.01$).
- Asthma-related hospitalization rates were low and similar across groups (3 in the low-dose budesonide/placebo group, 1 in the low-dose budesonide/formoterol, 5 in the high-dose budesonide/placebo group, and 2 in the high-dose budesonide/formoterol group).

STUDY CONCLUSIONS

The addition of formoterol to inhaled budesonide decreases mild and severe asthma exacerbations with better symptom control.

COMMENTARY

FACET showed that the addition of a LABA to ICS therapy reduced the rate of exacerbations and improved symptom control without increasing rates of adverse effects. A limitation was the presence of an induction period on an exceedingly high dose of inhaled budesonide not commonly used in regular practice. Importantly, the SMART trial[1] subsequently showed that LABA use was associated with an increased risk of death, particularly if used without an ICS. As a result, the US FDA placed a black-box warning on LABA and LABA+ICS products, and has requested that LABA manufacturers conduct 4 randomized controlled trials enrolling a total of 40,000 patients. AUSTRI,[2] the first such trial, has reported reassuring results. The 2007 National Asthma Education and Prevention Program guidelines recommend adding a LABA to ICS therapy in symptomatic patients with moderate or severe asthma as part of step-up therapy, and avoiding the use of LABAs alone.

Question

Is it reasonable to add a LABA to the regimen of patients with moderate or severe, persistent symptomatic asthma who are already on an ICS?

Answer

Yes, adding a LABA to an ICS for these patients leads to a reduction in symptoms and exacerbations.

References

1. Nelson HS, Weiss ST, Bleecker ER, Yancey SW, Dorinsky PM; SMART Study Group. The Salmeterol Multicenter Asthma Research Trial: A comparison of usual pharmacotherapy for asthma or usual pharmacotherapy plus salmeterol. *Chest.* 2006;129(1):15–26.
2. Stempel DA, Raphiou IH, Kral KM, et al; AUSTRI Investigators. Serious asthma events with fluticasone plus salmeterol versus fluticasone alone. *N Engl J Med.* 2016;374(19):1822–1830.

CHAPTER 93

TARGETING MOLECULAR DEFECTS IN CYSTIC FIBROSIS

Jessica Lee-Pancoast

A CFTR Potentiator in Patients With Cystic Fibrosis and the G551D Mutation

Ramsey BW, Davies J, McElvaney NG, et al. *N Engl J Med.* 2011;365(18):1663–1672

BACKGROUND

Prior to this study, all cystic fibrosis (CF) therapies treated downstream effects of the pathologic CFTR channel on various organ systems. The most common CFTR mutation is *Phe508del*, which leads to fewer (and somewhat dysfunctional) CFTR proteins at the cell surface. A minority carry the *G551D* mutation, which leads to a much less functional channel. Ivacaftor potentiates the CFTR channel by keeping it open for a longer duration.

OBJECTIVES

To determine efficacy and safety of ivacaftor in CF patients with at least 1 *G551D* mutation.

METHODS

Randomized, double-blind, placebo-controlled trial in North America, Europe, and Australia from 2009 to 2011.

Patients

161 patients with CF. Inclusion criteria included at least 1 *G551D* mutation allele, age ≥12 years, and FEV_1 40% to 90% of predicted value.

Interventions

Ivacaftor (150 mg twice daily) versus placebo for 48 weeks.

Outcomes

The primary outcome was absolute change from baseline in percent of predicted FEV_1 at week 24. Other outcomes included change in percent of predicted FEV_1 at week 48, respiratory symptom score, weight change from baseline, pulmonary exacerbations, and change in sweat chloride concentration (an indicator of CFTR function) from baseline.

KEY RESULTS

- At week 24, change in percent of predicted FEV_1 was greater in the ivacaftor group (10.4 percentage point improvement vs. 0.2 percentage point decrease, $p < 0.001$). This effect was first apparent at day 15 ($p < 0.001$), and was sustained through week 48 ($p < 0.001$).

- At 48 weeks, patients receiving ivacaftor had greater improvement from baseline symptom scores ($p < 0.001$) and were less likely to have had a pulmonary exacerbation (HR 0.46, $p = 0.001$).
- Ivacaftor patients gained an average of 2.7 kg more than placebo patients by 48 weeks ($p < 0.001$).
- At week 24, mean sweat chloride concentration was lower (indicating better CFTR function) in the ivacaftor group ($p < 0.001$) and below the diagnostic level for CF.
- Serious adverse events, mostly pulmonary exacerbations and hemoptysis, occurred more frequently in the placebo group (42% vs. 24%, p value not reported).

STUDY CONCLUSIONS

Ivacaftor was associated with improvements in lung function, risk of pulmonary exacerbations, respiratory symptoms, weight, and sweat chloride concentration.

COMMENTARY

While the *G551D* mutation is present in only 5% of CF patients, this trial was momentous both for the extent of clinical benefit demonstrated and for targeting molecular defects rather than symptoms – an approach that holds the potential to fundamentally transform the management and clinical course of CF. Although ivacaftor alone is not effective for those with the *Phe508del* mutation – likely because its mechanism of action (channel potentiation) is inadequate on its own when CFTR is infrequently present at the membrane – the combination of ivacaftor and lumacaftor (an agent that corrects CFTR misprocessing and increases its presence at the cell surface) demonstrates modest beneficial effects. The 2013 Cystic Fibrosis Foundation guidelines on chronic medications for maintenance of lung health now strongly recommend all patients over 6 years old with the *G551D* mutation be treated with ivacaftor.

Question

Should adult CF patients with *G551D* mutation receive ivacaftor?

Answer

Yes, ivacaftor is safe and improves outcomes in these patients.

CHAPTER 94

PIRFENIDONE IN IPF: THE ASCEND TRIAL

Neelam A. Phadke

A Phase 3 Trial of Pirfenidone in Patients With Idiopathic Pulmonary Fibrosis

King TE Jr, Bradford WZ, Castro-Bernardini S, et al. *N Engl J Med.* 2014;370(22): 2083–2092

BACKGROUND

By the time of this study, 3 multinational phase 3 trials had been conducted to assess whether pirfenidone, a novel oral antifibrosis agent, could improve survival and symptoms in patients with idiopathic pulmonary fibrosis (IPF). Given their predominantly positive – but inconsistent – results, pirfenidone was approved for use in Europe. However, the Food and Drug Administration (FDA) required a fourth randomized trial for approval in the United States, leading to this larger study with a much more strictly defined population of IPF patients.

OBJECTIVES

To determine the effect of pirfenidone on IPF progression.

METHODS

Randomized, double-blind, placebo-controlled trial at 127 sites in 9 countries on 5 continents from 2011 to 2013.

Patients

555 patients. Inclusion criteria included age 40 to 80 years, confirmed IPF (definite interstitial pneumonia on high-resolution CT or surgical lung biopsy confirmation) with FVC 50% to 90% predicted, DLCO 30% to 90% predicted, $FEV_1/FVC \geq 0.8$, and 6-minute walk distance ≥ 150 m. Exclusion criteria included active or recent smoking (within 3 months), history of asthma/COPD, connective tissue disease, known explanation for interstitial lung disease (e.g., radiation, sarcoidosis, infection, and malignancy), and previous exposure leading to pulmonary fibrosis.

Interventions

Oral pirfenidone (2,403 mg daily) versus placebo.

Outcomes

The primary outcome was death or $\geq 10\%$ decline in FVC at week 52. Secondary outcomes included 6-minute walk distance, progression-free survival, dyspnea (using self-reported questionnaires), IPF-related mortality, and all-cause mortality.

KEY RESULTS

- Fewer patients in the pirfenidone group died or had ≥10% FVC decline at 52 weeks (16.5% vs. 31.8%, $p < 0.001$).
- Mean decline from baseline FVC at 52 weeks was smaller in the pirfenidone group (235 mL vs. 428 mL, $p < 0.001$).
- Pirfenidone reduced the risk of death or disease progression (HR 0.57, 95% CI, 0.43–0.77, $p < 0.001$).
- There were no statistically significant differences between groups in dyspnea scores (29.1% vs. 36.1%, $p = 0.16$), death from IPF (1.1% vs. 2.5%, $p = 0.23$), and all-cause mortality (4.0% vs. 7.2%, $p = 0.10$).

STUDY CONCLUSIONS

Treatment with pirfenidone significantly reduced disease progression in patients with IPF.

COMMENTARY

ASCEND confirmed and extended the findings from 2 of 3 prior studies. In particular, its strict enrollment of only those with complete pulmonary function tests and either a biopsy or CT scan consistent with IPF was an improvement from previous studies. The main caveat is the trial's short follow-up time. As a result of ASCEND, pirfenidone was promptly approved by the FDA. Along with nintedanib, a novel tyrosine kinase inhibitor approved shortly thereafter, pirfenidone remains the only targeted IPF therapy available. Given the associated improvements in functional activity and the apparent absence of harm, the 2015 American Thoracic Society IPF treatment guidelines conditionally recommend pirfenidone or nintedanib at the discretion of the patient and treating provider. Long-term follow-up and combination therapy trials are ongoing.

Question

Is it reasonable to treat patients with IPF using pirfenidone?

Answer

Yes, pirfenidone can reduce disease progression (as defined by decline in FVC and 6-minute walk distance), although it has not been shown to significantly improve symptoms or short-term mortality.

CHAPTER 95

ANTIBIOTICS IN COPD EXACERBATIONS

Mounica Vallurupalli

Antibiotic Therapy in Exacerbations of Chronic Obstructive Pulmonary Disease

Anthonisen NR, Manfreda J, Warren CP, Hershfield ES, Harding GK, Nelson NA. *Ann Intern Med.* 1987;106(2):196–204

BACKGROUND

At the time of this study, treatment for chronic obstructive pulmonary disease (COPD) exacerbations was not fully standardized, but it was generally believed that management of bacterial colonization or infection played a role. Antibiotics were frequently used in these situations, but there was neither a standard definition for COPD exacerbations nor high-quality evidence to support this practice.

OBJECTIVES

To identify the effects of broad-spectrum antibiotic therapy in COPD exacerbations.

METHODS

Randomized, double-blind, crossover trial.

Patients

173 patients. Inclusion criteria included age ≥35 years, diagnosis of COPD, FEV_1 <70% predicted that did not increase to ≥80% with bronchodilators, and TLC >80% predicted. Exclusion criteria included congestive heart failure, cancer, stroke, or disorders requiring antibiotic therapy. Additionally, exacerbations were excluded if treating physicians felt patients were too ill to be randomized.

Interventions

Antibiotics (trimethoprim-sulfamethoxazole, doxycycline, or amoxicillin) versus placebo for 10 days for the first exacerbation. Subsequent exacerbations were treated in a crossover manner with alternating antibiotic treatment or placebo. Between exacerbations, all patients received inhaled albuterol and oral theophylline; some received prednisone 5 to 10 mg daily. Some patients received higher doses of steroids during exacerbations.

Outcomes

The primary outcome was treatment success of exacerbations (defined as resolution of symptoms within 21 days of the exacerbation assessed by a disease-specific questionnaire). Exacerbations were defined as a combination of 3 cardinal symptoms – increased dyspnea, sputum volume, and sputum purulence – and categorized based on the number of these symptoms: type 1 (all 3 symptoms), type 2 (2 symptoms), or type 3 (1 symptom and other minor clinical criteria). Secondary outcomes included number of exacerbations, exacerbation category, persistence of any symptom at 21 days, and deterioration (need for hospitalization or unblinded antibiotic therapy within the 21-day follow-up period).

KEY RESULTS

- The treatment success rate was higher in the antibiotic group (68.1% vs. 55.0%, $p < 0.01$).
- Rate of deterioration was higher in the placebo group (18.9% vs. 9.9%, $p < 0.05$).
- Treatment success rate was higher in type 1 exacerbations treated with antibiotics compared to those treated with placebo (62.9% vs. 43.0%, no p value reported).
- Of 448 total exacerbations, 86 were not treated according to the study protocol, including 35 cases in which patients were deemed too ill to be randomized.

STUDY CONCLUSIONS

Compared to placebo, antibiotics increase the rate of resolution of COPD exacerbations and prevent clinical deterioration.

COMMENTARY

This study introduced a way to define the presence and severity of COPD exacerbations using patient-reported symptoms of dyspnea, sputum purulence, and sputum volume. Many subsequent studies, as well as the Global Initiative for Chronic Obstructive Lung Disease (GOLD) guidelines, have adopted these symptoms to define COPD exacerbations. While COPD exacerbation treatment regimens have evolved significantly since this trial, it was the first to show that patients with these cardinal symptoms benefit from antibiotic therapy. Limitations include significant subject drop out, steroid use by an unknown proportion of participants, and many exacerbations treated outside of the study protocol. Some advocate treatment with antibiotics in the setting of 2 out of 3 of these cardinal symptoms, and the 2016 GOLD guidelines recommend antibiotics in patients with all 3.

Question

Should patients with a diagnosis of COPD and increased sputum, sputum purulence, and dyspnea receive antibiotics?

Answer

Yes, antibiotic therapy may reduce symptoms for patients with COPD exacerbation.

RHEUMATOLOGY

CHAPTER 96

ANTI-TNFα THERAPY IN RHEUMATOID ARTHRITIS

Alexandra Charrow

Randomised Double-Blind Comparison of Chimeric Monoclonal Antibody to Tumour Necrosis Factor Alpha (cA2) Versus Placebo in Rheumatoid Arthritis

Elliott MJ, Maini RN, Feldmann M, et al. *Lancet.* 1994;344(8930):1105–1110

BACKGROUND

Rheumatoid arthritis (RA) is sometimes refractory to traditional disease-modifying antirheumatic disease drug (DMARD) therapy. Prior to this study, tumor necrosis factor α (TNFα) had been identified as a mediator of inflammation in RA and therefore a potential prime target for specific immunotherapy. However, while beneficial responses had been observed in patients after open-label administration, definitive, blinded, randomized data were lacking.

OBJECTIVES

To confirm the efficacy and safety of chimeric monoclonal antibody to TNFα (cA2) and the role of TNFα in the inflammatory dysregulation of RA.

METHODS

Randomized, double-blind trial in 4 European centers.

Patients

72 patients whose RA medications, including other DMARDs, were stopped. Inclusion criteria included meeting the American College of Rheumatology criteria for RA for ≥6 months, active disease, history of failed treatment with ≥1 DMARD, and evidence of erosive arthritis on hand and foot radiography. Exclusion criteria included severe physical incapacity, joint ankylosis, severe complete blood count anomalies, active pathology on chest film, and history of cancer or HIV.

Interventions

Low-dose cA2 (one infusion dosed at 1 mg/kg) versus high-dose cA2 (one infusion dosed at 10 mg/kg) versus placebo (one infusion of sterile saline).

Outcomes

The primary outcome was response at 4 weeks (defined by a 20% response in the Paulus index, which incorporates improvements in duration of morning stiffness, tender-joint and swollen-joint score, patient and observer assessment of disease severity, and ESR). Secondary outcomes included pain score and grip strength, and adverse events included cardiovascular, respiratory, and musculoskeletal symptoms.

KEY RESULTS

- 2/24 placebo recipients achieved response, compared to 11/25 of low-dose cA2 recipients ($p = 0.0083$) and 19/24 high-dose cA2 recipients ($p < 0.0001$).
- More patients receiving high-dose cA2 achieved 50% index improvement compared to those receiving placebo (58% vs. 8%, $p = 0.0005$).
- 68% of adverse events occurred in those receiving cA2, with infections being the most common type; 2/72 patients experienced severe adverse events (probable pneumonia and pathologic clavicular fracture).

STUDY CONCLUSIONS

Blockade of TNFα with cA2 is effective and safe in the short-term treatment of RA.

COMMENTARY

This trial was the first to provide blinded, randomized evidence for the use of a TNFα antibody in the treatment of a rheumatologic condition. Caveats include small sample size and comparison to placebo rather than other DMARDs. Along with those from subsequent evaluations combining TNFα antibody and DMARD therapy, these study findings are reflected in the 2015 American College of Rheumatology RA treatment guidelines, which recommend TNFα antibody medications as part of most treatment strategies for patients with refractory RA or those requiring combination therapy. Over 20 years later, TNFα antibody therapy is now used in a number of conditions ranging from RA to psoriatic arthritis to inflammatory bowel disease.

Question

Is it reasonable to consider TNFα antibody therapy for patients with RA?

Answer

Yes, it can be used to achieve response among patients with disease that is refractory to traditional DMARD therapy or select patients who require combination therapy.

CHAPTER 97

TREATMENT OF ANCA-ASSOCIATED VASCULITIS: THE RAVE TRIAL

Alexandra Charrow

Rituximab Versus Cyclophosphamide for ANCA-Associated Vasculitis

Stone JH, Merkel PA, Spiera R, et al. *N Engl J Med.* 2010;363(3):221–232

BACKGROUND

For 40 years, cyclophosphamide and concomitant steroids had been the standard of care for halting disease progression and decreasing morbidity among patients with ANCA-associated vasculitis (AAV). However, cyclophosphamide has significant toxicities including malignancy, infection, and cytopenias. Chronic steroid use is also associated with significant side effects. Studies had suggested that rituximab was effective and safer than cyclophosphamide-based regimens, but no randomized controlled trials had compared their safety and efficacy.

OBJECTIVES

To demonstrate noninferiority of rituximab therapy compared to standard cyclophosphamide therapy for the induction of complete remission in severe AAV.

METHODS

Randomized, double-blind, double-dummy, noninferiority trial at 9 centers between 2004 and 2008.

Patients

197 patients. Inclusion criteria included AAV confirmed by positive serum assays for proteinase 3-ANCA or myeloperoxidase-ANCA, manifestations of severe disease, and a Birmingham Vasculitis Activity Score for Wegener's Granulomatosis (BVAS/WG) ≥3. Exclusion criteria included history of Churg–Strauss or antiglomerular basement membrane disease, active infection, malignancy, hepatitis B or C, and HIV infection.

Interventions

Intravenous rituximab (375 mg/m^2 weekly for 4 weeks) plus placebo-cyclophosphamide versus cyclophosphamide (2 mg/kg daily) plus placebo-rituximab. All patients received pulses of methylprednisolone followed by prednisone tapered off at 5 months if disease-free.

Outcomes

The primary outcome was steroid-free remission (defined by a BVAS/WG of 0 and successful taper of prednisone) at 6 months. Secondary outcomes included rates of disease flare (defined by an increase in BVAS/WG score of >1 point), cumulative steroid use, BVAS/WG score of 0 on ≤10-mg prednisone daily, and adverse event rates.

KEY RESULTS

- Similar proportions of patients in the rituximab and cyclophosphamide groups achieved steroid-free remission (64% vs. 53%, $p < 0.001$ at the prespecified noninferiority margin).
- In relapsing disease, those receiving rituximab also achieved remission without prednisone more frequently (67% vs. 42%, $p = 0.01$).
- Patients in the rituximab group achieved ANCA-negativity more frequently (47% vs. 24%, $p = 0.004$) and experienced fewer adverse events (33% vs. 22%, $p = 0.01$).

STUDY CONCLUSIONS

Rituximab therapy was not inferior to daily cyclophosphamide treatment for induction of remission in severe AAV and may be superior in relapsing disease.

COMMENTARY

RAVE was groundbreaking in demonstrating the efficacy of an alternative to cyclophosphamide. Study caveats include exclusion of certain subgroups (e.g., those with ANCA-negative disease) and administration of steroids for much of the follow-up period. In addition, while a contemporary study reported 12-month remission among those receiving several doses of intravenous cyclophosphamide along with rituximab,[1] patients randomized to rituximab in RAVE did not receive any cyclophosphamide. While longer-term follow-up data are needed to clarify optimal regimens, the RAVE findings have informed the 2014 British Society for Rheumatology guidelines, which list rituximab alongside cyclophosphamide as the 2 mainstay options in the treatment of severe AAV.

Question

Is it reasonable to use rituximab for the treatment of AAV?

Answer

Yes, rituximab represents a noninferior alternative to cyclophosphamide therapy and may even be superior in the treatment of relapsing disease.

References

1. Jones RB, Tervaert JW, Hauser T, et al; European Vasculitis Study Group. Rituximab versus cyclophosphamide in ANCA-associated renal vasculitis. *N Engl J Med.* 2010;363:211–220.

CHAPTER 98

HYDROXYCHLOROQUINE IN SLE

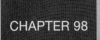

Alexandra Charrow

A Randomized Study of the Effect of Withdrawing Hydroxychloroquine Sulfate in Systemic Lupus Erythematosus

The Canadian Hydroxychloroquine Study Group. *N Engl J Med.* 1991;324(3):150–154

BACKGROUND

Prior to this study, antimalarial drugs such as hydroxychloroquine were believed to have the potential to limit symptoms and manifestations associated with systemic lupus erythematosus (SLE) as well as reduce the need for, and long-term side effects of, glucocorticoids. Due to a lack of definitive, prospective evidence about benefit and safety, however, clinicians were reluctant to utilize these agents for long-term disease control.

OBJECTIVES

To evaluate the effect of hydroxychloroquine on clinical flares in patients with quiescent SLE.

METHODS

Randomized, double-blind, placebo-controlled trial in 5 Canadian hospitals between 1986 and 1987.

Patients

47 patients with SLE. Inclusion criteria included existing treatment with hydroxychloroquine (100 to 400 mg daily) for ≥6 months and clinically stable disease for ≥3 months. Exclusion criteria included age <16 years old, hydroxychloroquine dosages >6.5 mg/kg/day, retinopathy, and comorbidities that might compromise patient health from an SLE flare.

Interventions

Hydroxychloroquine (at existing dose) versus placebo (discontinuation of hydroxychloroquine without taper). Ten patients in each group also received prednisone. Patients were followed for 24 weeks.

Outcomes

The primary outcome was time to SLE flare (defined as increased disease severity or development of disease-related manifestations, including alopecia, cutaneous vasculitis, lymphadenopathy, pleuritis, pericarditis, arthritis, or constitutional symptoms). Secondary outcomes included a required change in prednisone dose or severe exacerbation of disease (determined by investigator judgment or development of vasculitis, myositis, active glomerulonephritis, or nervous system manifestations).

KEY RESULTS

- 16/22 patients in the placebo group experienced SLE flares compared to 9/25 in the hydroxychloroquine group (RR 2.5, 95% CI 1.08–5.58, $p = 0.02$).
- 5/22 patients in the placebo group developed severe exacerbation of disease compared to 1/25 in the hydroxychloroquine group (RR 6.1, 95% CI 0.72–52.44, $p = 0.06$).
- No patients required decreases or discontinuation of hydroxychloroquine due to adverse events.
- There were no statistically significant differences between groups in the change in prednisone dose ($p = 0.27$).

STUDY CONCLUSIONS

Patients with quiescent SLE on hydroxychloroquine are less likely to have a clinical flare if continued on the medication.

COMMENTARY

While other agents (e.g., steroids and cyclophosphamide) were available for treating SLE flares, this trial was the first to prospectively demonstrate the role of a long-term steroid-sparing medication in preventing flares in patients with quiescent disease. Caveats include the approach to defining flares (weighing all organ system reactions, from proteinuria to rash, equally) and shorter follow-up period than potentially needed to observe flares or allow for full clearance of hydroxychloroquine. Along with other work demonstrating hydroxychloroquine's safety and broad benefit in SLE, the findings from this study have contributed to the widespread practice and convention of initiating the medication in all SLE patients for whom there are no contraindications.

Question

Should extended hydroxychloroquine be considered in the treatment of patients with SLE?

Answer

Yes, the medication can prevent clinical flares and should be considered in all patients for whom there is no contraindication to its use.

CHAPTER 99

TREATMENT STRATEGIES IN RA: THE BeSt STUDY

Alexandra Charrow

Clinical and Radiographic Outcomes of Four Different Treatment Strategies in Patients With Early Rheumatoid Arthritis (the BeSt Study): A Randomized, Controlled Trial

Goekoop-Ruiterman YP, de Vries-Bouwstra JK, Allaart CF, et al. *Arthritis Rheum.* 2005;52(11):3381–3390

BACKGROUND

In the decades preceding this study, there had been a significant increase in effective disease-modifying antirheumatic drugs (DMARDs) available for the treatment of RA, including infliximab, methotrexate (MTX), sulfasalazine, cyclosporine A, and hydroxychloroquine. However, despite the development and investigation of such agents, the optimal therapeutic algorithm for preventing long-term joint dysfunction and damage was unknown.

OBJECTIVES

To determine the most effective treatment strategy for reducing joint dysfunction and damage in early RA.

METHODS

Randomized, controlled, double-blind trial in 20 centers in the Netherlands between 2000 and 2002.

Patients

508 patients. Inclusion criteria included early RA with duration <2 years, age >18 years, and active disease (>6 of 66 swollen joints, >6 of 68 tender joints, and elevated ESR or global health score of >20 mm/100 mm on visual analog scale). Exclusion criteria included previous DMARD treatment, history of malignancy, and substance abuse.

Interventions

Participants were randomized to 1 of 4 treatments: sequential monotherapy (group 1: MTX, replaced by more aggressive monotherapy if no initial response) versus step-up combination therapy (group 2: MTX, with other agents added if no initial response) versus initial combination therapy with prednisone (group 3: tapered high-dose prednisone along with MTX and sulfasalazine, with DMARDs replaced if no response) versus initial combination therapy with infliximab (group 4: MTX and infliximab, with replacement of both if no response). Adequate disease suppression was defined as a Disease Activity Score in 44 joints score of ≤2.4.

Outcomes

Improvement in functional ability (≥0.2 decrease in Dutch Health Assessment Questionnaire score [D-HAQ]) and improvement in radiographic disease (>20% decrease in modified Sharp/Van der Heijde Score).

KEY RESULTS
- Compared to other groups, groups 3 and 4 demonstrated earlier functional improvement (mean D-HAQ scores 0.6 vs. 1.0 in groups 1 and 2, $p < 0.001$) that began at 3 months and persisted through 1 year.
- Groups 3 and 4 also displayed less radiographic disease (SHS scores 0.5 and 1.0, respectively vs. 2.0 and 2.5 for groups 1 and 2, $p < 0.001$).
- Greater than 40% of patients in groups 1 and 2 sustained adequate suppression with MTX monotherapy.

STUDY CONCLUSIONS
In those with early RA, initial combination therapy resulted in earlier functional improvement and less radiographic damage compared to DMARD monotherapy or step-up combination therapy.

COMMENTARY

BeSt informed the management of early RA. First, the considerable proportion of patients adequately controlled on DMARD monotherapy – along with the study's incomplete side-effect data and lack of focus on costs – bolstered guideline recommendations to initiate monotherapy in most patients. Second, it expanded the indications for early combination therapy by showing benefit in patients for whom more rapid resolution of joint symptoms is critical (e.g., for work-related activities).[1,2]

Question
Should all patients with symptomatic, early RA be treated with DMARD monotherapy?

Answer
No, while many patients are well controlled on monotherapy, combination therapy can lead to faster functional improvement in patients who require more rapid symptom resolution. However, these benefits should be weighed against the potential expense and side effects.

References
1. Singh JA, Saag KG, Bridges SL Jr, et al. 2015 American College of Rheumatology Guidelines for the Treatment of Rheumatoid Arthritis. *Arthritis Rheumatol.* 2016;68(1):1–26.
2. Smolen JS, Landewé R, Breedveld FC, et al. EULAR recommendations for the management of rheumatoid arthritis with synthetic and biological disease-modifying antirheumatic drugs: 2013 update. *Ann Rheum Dis.* 2014;73(3):492–509.

CHAPTER 100

INDUCTION TREATMENT FOR LUPUS NEPHRITIS: THE ALMS TRIAL

Alexandra Charrow

Mycophenolate Mofetil Versus Cyclophosphamide for Induction Treatment of Lupus Nephritis

Appel GB, Contreras G, Dooley MA, et al. *J Am Soc Nephrol.* 2009;20(5):1103–1112

BACKGROUND

Based on evidence accumulated over the 3 decades prior to this study, intravenous cyclophosphamide (IVC) had long been the mainstay for induction therapy in patients with lupus nephritis (LN). However, IVC also has major limitations, including slow response, incomplete disease control, and considerable toxicity risk. In contrast, small studies from single countries had shown that mycophenolate mofetil (MMF) could be as effective as IVC for induction with potential advantages and lower risk of toxicity. However, prospective evidence from large, multinational trials was lacking.

OBJECTIVES

To assess the efficacy and safety of MMF versus IVC as induction therapy for LN.

METHODS

Randomized, controlled, open-label trial in 88 centers across 20 countries between 2005 and 2006.[1]

Patients

370 patients. Inclusion criteria included age 12 to 75 years, SLE based on revised American College of Rheumatology criteria, long-term immunosuppression, and kidney biopsy within 6 months confirming class III–V LN. Exclusion criteria included dialysis for >2 weeks, kidney transplantation, immunodeficiency, substance abuse, malignancy, lymphoproliferative disease, and severe end-organ disease.

Interventions

24 weeks of open-label oral MMF (0.5 g twice daily, titrated to target dose of 3 g/day) versus IVC (0.75 g/m^2 monthly, titrated to maintain leukocyte nadir between 2,500 and 4,000/mm^3). All patients received concomitant corticosteroid therapy.

Outcomes

The primary outcome was treatment response after 24 weeks, defined as stabilization/improvement in serum creatinine and decrease in proteinuria (urine protein/creatinine ratio <3 in those with nephrotic-range proteinuria; >50% reduction in those with subnephrotic-range proteinuria). Secondary outcomes included complete renal remission, systemic disease activity, and adverse events.

KEY RESULTS

- There were no statistically significant differences in treatment response rates between MMF and IVC groups (56.2% vs. 53.0%, $p = 0.58$).
- MMF led to treatment response more frequently among black and mixed-race (60.4% vs. 38.5%, $p = 0.033$) and Hispanic (60.9% vs. 38.8%, $p = 0.011$) patients.
- There were no statistically significant differences in rates of complete renal remission, systemic disease activity, or adverse events (including serious adverse events and infections) between groups.

STUDY CONCLUSIONS

MMF was not superior to IVC as induction treatment for LN.

COMMENTARY

In contrast to preceding studies, ALMS did not demonstrate the overall superiority of MMF over IVC in the induction treatment of LN. However, MMF appeared more efficacious among certain ethnic subgroups. Study caveats include lack of blinding and the potential influence of the open-label design on event reporting. The ALMS findings are reflected in LN treatment guidelines, which suggest that MMF and IVC are equivalent for induction therapy, but that IVC may be less effective in black and Hispanic populations.[2]

Question

Is there a universally preferred agent for induction therapy among patients with proteinuria and class III–V LN?

Answer

No, MMF and IVC are equivalent therapies for induction overall, but individual factors should be considered, as MMF may be more effective in certain subgroups.

References

1. Sinclair A, Appel G, Dooley MA, et al. Mycophenolate mofetil as induction and maintenance therapy for lupus nephritis: Rationale and protocol for the randomized, controlled Aspreva Lupus Management Study (ALMS). *Lupus*. 2007;16(12):972–980.
2. Hahn BH, McMahon MA, Wilkinson A, et al; American College of Rheumatology. American College of Rheumatology guidelines for screening, treatment, and management of lupus nephritis. *Arthritis Care Res (Hoboken)*. 2012;64(6):797–808.

INDEX